# Interpersonal Skills for Nurses and Health Care Professionals

### R.F. Wondrak

**Blackwell
Science**

© 1998 by
Blackwell Science Ltd
Editorial Offices:
Osney Mead, Oxford OX2 0EL
25 John Street, London WC1N 2BL
23 Ainslie Place, Edinburgh EH3 6AJ
350 Main Street, Malden
 MA 02148 5018, USA
54 University Street, Carlton
 Victoria 3053, Australia
10, rue Casimir Delavigne
 75006 Paris, France

Other Editorial Offices:

Blackwell Wissenschafts-Verlag GmbH
Kurfürstendamm 57
10707 Berlin, Germany

Blackwell Science KK
MG Kodenmacho Building
7–10 Kodenmacho Nihombashi
Chuo-ku, Tokyo 104, Japan

Iowa State University Press
A Blackwell Science Company
2121 S. State Avenue
Ames, Iowa 50014-8300, USA

First published 1998
Reprinted 2001

Set by DP Photosetting, Aylesbury, Bucks
Printed and bound in Great Britain
by MPG Books Ltd, Bodmin, Cornwall

DISTRIBUTORS

Marston Book Services Ltd
PO Box 269
Abingdon
Oxon OX14 4YN
(*Orders:* Tel: 01235 465500
        Fax: 01235 465555)

USA
Blackwell Science, Inc.
Commerce Place
350 Main Street
Malden, MA 02148 5018
(*Orders:* Tel:  800 759 6102
           781 388 8250
      Fax: 781 388 8255)

Canada
Login Brothers Book Company
324 Saulteaux Crescent
Winnipeg, Manitoba R3J 3T2
(*Orders:* Tel: 204 224 4068)

Australia
Blackwell Science Pty Ltd
54 University Street
Carlton, Victoria 3053
(*Orders:* Tel:  03 9347 0300
      Fax: 03 9347 5001)

A catalogue record for this title
is available from the British Library

ISBN 0-632-04144-7

Wondrak, R. F. (Robert F.)
    Interpersonal skills for nurses and health care
professionals / R. F. Wondrak
        p.      cm.
Includes bibliographical references and index.
ISBN 0-632-04144-7
    1. Communication in nursing. 2. Interpersonal
communication. 3. Nurse and patient.
4. Interpersonal relations. I. Title.
    [DNLM: 1. Interpersonal Relations nurses'
instruction. 2. Nursing Care—pschology.
3. Attitude of Health Personnel. WY 87W8725i
1998]
RT23.W66   1998
610.73'01,4—dc21
DNLM/DLC
for Library of Congress                    98–25010
                                              CIP

For further information on Blackwell Science,
visit our website:
www.blackwell-science.com

# Contents

*Foreword*     v

*Preface*     vi

*Acknowledgements*     x

1   The Interpersonal Arena     1

2   Theoretical Approaches     9

3   Approaches to the Care of the Child     32

4   Approaches to Care in Adolescence     61

5   Approaches to the Care of the Adult     85

6   Approaches to the Care of the Older Patient     105

7   Approaches to the Care of the Adult with Mental
Health Disorder     125

8   Approaches to Cultural and Spiritual Care     148

9   Conclusions: An Eclectic Approach     161

*Index*     164

# Foreword

Communicating clearly with people is one of the most difficult skills we struggle to acquire in life. Some people seem to have a natural ability to get on with others, to convey ideas, to empathise, to support and to empower, whilst others of us feel that such skills do not come easily. Yet interpersonal skills are central to the work of health care professionals as well as central to our being able to function as citizens, partners and parents. Working with others demands that we are able to understand different perspectives, to spot misunderstandings and detect clues as to why we behave as we do. Fortunately we do not have to rely on being born with such skills, we can acquire them by study and by practice. Indeed, good interpersonal skills are very rarely the product of nature alone. They need to be nurtured and developed every bit as much as good practical or academic skills.

There has probably never been a time when it has been as important as it is today that health care professionals develop these skills. We know that people's illness and suffering is intimately connected with their perception of the world they inhabit, with the way in which they view themselves and others, and with the frame of mind within which they interpret what happens to them. To be able to communicate and understand is a long way towards being able to help and support. It is also vital that health care professionals who work in teams understand other team members and their professional worlds so that, together, they can maximise their effectiveness.

Rob Wondrak's book is intended to enable students and professionals to develop the interpersonal skills they need in their everyday work. It makes clear the importance of these skills to the care of children, adolescents and adults, and emphasises the cultural and spiritual dimensions of good interpersonal skills. These are skills which none of the helping professions can afford to be without.

*Professor Linda Challis*
*Pro-Vice Chancellor and Head of Health Care*
*Oxford Brookes University*

# Preface

This book attempts to bring together many of the themes from a wide variety of texts already available on the subject of interpersonal skills for nurses and health care workers.

In doing so it seeks to address what is considered to be a gap in the introductory texts available for nurses undertaking Project 2000 courses and health care workers involved in the process of caring for patients in a clinical setting.

This text provides a multi-professional commentary, considering the care of patients/clients from the differing perspectives of a range of health care workers. Increasingly the importance of multi-professional understanding and education is being seen as the most effective way to develop practice for the new millennium. All the care workers represented in this book collaborate in the delivery of care, and there is a need to understand each other's role in a much clearer way. This book offers a contribution to this process.

The current texts on interpersonal skills fall into three main groups. First, there are the more academically orientated which primarily focus on theoretical aspects of interpersonal psychology and social psychology.

Then there is a wide range which focuses more on the practical aspects, for example books which consist of exercises and workbook-type texts.

More recently books on interpersonal skills have appeared which attempt to apply some of the main implications of theory and research into the domain of nursing and health care.

When surveying the large number of volumes already available, what seemed to be missing was a more straightforward introductory text which attempted to examine the experience of a range of carers working in health care settings, and to link these to common theoretical approaches. Thus interpersonal knowledge and skills are related to what is often experienced in the carers' initial period of practice.

A 'life-span' approach is taken, providing the reader with the ability to follow through potential events that contribute to a person's life. Thus the book begins by exploring three main theoretical ideas – the psychodynamic approach, the behavioural approach and the person-centred approach – and relates these to the life periods of childhood, adolescence, adulthood and old age.

Moreover, in addition to this approach, the book focuses upon three areas which transcend the life-span. These are cultural and spiritual issues, and a more in-depth discussion of mental health issues. This is because there are valid criticisms of a direct 'life-span' approach, suggesting that while this approach offers 'neat and orderly' sequences to life, research has often demonstrated the absence of strongly age-linked periods (Bee, 1994).

The book is also aimed to serve as a refresher for many health workers engaged in clinical practice who wish to invigorate awareness of their day-to-day experience, with theoretical considerations which remain central to the way they work. Each chapter will begin with a short account by a health care professional of her own experiences at the beginning of her career.

This is an attempt to sharpen the text and make it more readable by allowing the reader to identify with the personal account of a practitioner. This brief 'reflective' account is often a much more open way of communicating and learning about practice.

## Rationale for the book

The available research indicates that interpersonal skills are not being transposed into clinical situations.

This has been recognised for many years; for example MacLeod-Clark (1985) argues that while social scientists have been exploring the area of communication and interpersonal skills, particularly in nursing, for at least two decades, there has been little apparent impact upon professional practice. While there are several explanations for this (Bannister and Kagan, 1985; Davidson, 1985; Faulkner, 1985; Kagan, 1985; MacLeod-Clark, 1985), one possible reason is that knowledge and awareness of communication and interpersonal skills have been disconnected from what workers actually feel when they are in clinical settings. It is now timely to attempt to bring together key themes and relate these to what the practitioner actually does in day-to-day practice.

The book will explore theories underlying the development of interpersonal skills and these will be developed as themes. Kagan (1985) has reminded us about the assumptions which lie behind the skills approach to improving interpersonal behaviour. Here she argues that particularly in the UK, social skills training has grown out of a model of social interaction first studied by social psychologists such as Michael Argyle (Argyle, 1994). This approach was stimulated by a growth in ergonomics, or person–machine interactions. This particular approach has been criticised by later writers for being too mechanistic (Morse and Johnson, 1991).

These criticisms were mainly fuelled by the humanistic approach to the understanding of human behaviour from writers such as Rogers (1961) and more lately in the arena of interpersonal and communication skills (Heron, 1973, 1990).

Currently the scene is very confusing. Part of the problem for this is that interpersonal skills are often referred to synonymously as communication skills, social skills, counselling skills or therapeutic skills and thus the student who is attempting to understand the links between available theory and the relevance for their own practice becomes confused by the myriad of terms relating to the area. This is addressed by exploring approaches to human interaction and their relevance to practice.

## Notes to the reader

The term 'health worker' or 'carer' is used extensively throughout to represent any health care professional, be they nurse, doctor, physiotherapist, occupational therapist or other paramedical discipline. The book will also be of assistance to any student undertaking a health-related course of study in interpersonal skills.

Rather than referring to 'he/she', all references to carers in this book are addressed as 'she'. The patient/client will be simply referred to as 'he' at appropriate points in the text. The aim is for this to be a short-hand convention to simplify the process of description.

Attempts have been made throughout the book to keep the examples as relevant to clinical practice as possible, with regular 'clinical case' accounts.

Also where relevant, further sources of reading have been offered at the end of each chapter.

*Robert Wondrak*

# References

Argyle, M. (1994) *The Psychology of Interpersonal Behaviour*, 5th edn. Penguin Books, London.

Bannister, P. and Kagan, C. (1985) The need for research into interpersonal skills in nursing. In *Interpersonal Skills in Nursing: Research and Applications* (C.M. Kagan, ed.), pp. 44–61. Chapman and Hall, London.

Bee, H. (1994) *Lifespan Development*. Harper Collins, New York.

Davidson, C. (1985) The theoretical antecedents to interpersonal skills training. In *Interpersonal Skills in Nursing: Research and Applications* (C.M. Kagan, ed.), pp. 22–44. Chapman and Hall, London.

Faulkner, A. (1985) The organisational context of interpersonal skills in nursing. In *Interpersonal Skills in Nursing: Research and Applications* (C.M. Kagan, ed.), pp. 65–76. Chapman and Hall, London.

Heron, J. (1973) *Experiential Training Techniques*. Human Potential Research Project, University of Surrey, Guildford.

Heron, J. (1990) *Client Practitioner Interventions*. Sage Books, London.

Macleod-Clark, J. (1985) The development of research in interpersonal skills in nursing. In *Interpersonal Skills in Nursing: Research and Applications* (C.M. Kagan, ed.), pp. 9–22. Chapman and Hall, London.

Morse, J.M. and Johnson, J.L. (1991) *The Illness Experience*. Sage Publications, California, USA.

Rogers, C.R. (1961) *On Becoming a Person: A Therapist's View of Psychotherapy*. Houghton Mifflin, Boston.

# Acknowledgements

I am grateful to all the people who have assisted me in the development of this book: to Sarah-Kate Powell and Griselda Campbell at Blackwell Science for their patience and encouragement, and to the reviewers, particularly André Le May, Sandy Oldfield and Jan Snowball.

The idea for this text came from the feedback of students and colleagues over the past few years. So I would like to thank the staff of the School of Health at the University of Western Sydney, Australia, especially Mavis Bickerton the Dean, and Esther Chang the Head of School.

Also to all my colleagues and students at Oxford Brookes University, UK.

Finally I would like to thank my family, Kath, Matthew and Victoria, for their love, support and understanding.

# Chapter 1
# The Interpersonal Arena

This chapter will explore the use of the term 'interpersonal skill', within the context of offering effective patient care. This means developing the skills of assessing how the patient's psychological needs are related to physical needs and how both of these are affected by spiritual needs.

The term 'interpersonal arena' may seem inappropriate at first. The term was used by Dryden (1984) to describe the variation and confusion within the counselling and therapy field, due to the number of approaches used by various therapists. It is used in this context to refer to the uncertainty created by a number of approaches to the application of interpersonal skills within health care practice.

For many carers, particularly at the beginning of their careers, there is a tension between being able to spend appropriate time getting to know the patient as an individual and the everyday workload demands. For the health worker embarking upon clinical practice for the first time, it may feel like an 'arena', with conflicting pressures to consider the *psychological*, *physical* and *spiritual* aspects of care. Despite the emphasis, in health literature, on 'holistic care' (which means combining these three elements together in the consideration of the patient's care, Fig. 1.1), it continues to be split into parts. This means that in the desire to offer effective care, with staff often under pressure, 'care' is separated, with only lip-service to regarding the individual as a 'whole' person (Fulford *et al.*, 1996).

This is an account of a first-year student nurse, Elizabeth, as she recalls commencing her nursing placement. The ward is an adult surgical care area in a large teaching hospital.

'I remember thinking back very clearly about my first experiences as I walked through the door of ward 15. I can recall powerful feelings of anxiety and also of excitement, the smell of polish, cooked cabbage, disinfectant. Everyone looked busy, all the staff seemed to know exactly what they were doing and I was left with a great feeling of

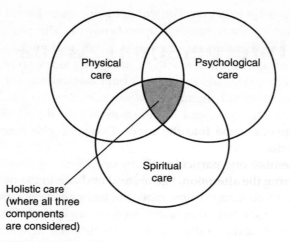

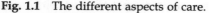

**Fig. 1.1** The different aspects of care.

inadequacy as I wondered how I could actually settle in to what seemed to me to be a place where everyone knew their role.

I recall the faces of the patients. They seemed to convey mixed moods and emotions, a strong mixture of cheerfulness by some people and pain and apathy in others. I remember being greeted by a staff nurse called Sandra, who took me to find the nurse in charge and then we obtained a key so that I could lock my possessions into a cupboard at the end of a ward. The key was returned to the nurse in charge. I remember feeling some irrational anxiety as my possessions were locked away, as if I was being separated from what little form of security I had at that moment.

I now recall these strange, bizarre feelings with some humour! The staff seemed friendly enough, there were smiles, but most people seemed to be too busy for anything more than a brief greeting.

The first "report handover" was terrible, me scribbling away, listening intently and trying to comprehend some of the terms being used to describe medical conditions. I remember my notes at the end of each session, having great gaps. The names of some patients not known. The general air of solemnity was too strong, and I did not feel confident enough to cause an interruption by asking questions which I thought might be perceived as facile.

I was allocated to a nurse called Margaret who was my mentor and remember attempting to stay as close as I could for the first few hours, so that I could try and feel as if I had something to do. I can clearly recall her being very busy, and I was left thinking I ought to find something else to get on with but not being quite sure. I recall feeling that I didn't want to impinge upon her work with patients. This was despite her friendliness, often asking me to come and help her. I remember at one point finding myself in a sideward trying to look busy; there was clearly much work but I was unaware of what needed to be done and had already asked several times. To ask again seemed to me foolish, so instead I attempted to tidy things and look busy when anyone came into the room. Everyone else seemed to know what to do.

I remember one particular afternoon where my mentor suggested that, during the afternoon, I go around and talk to the patients and get to know them better. I remember the feelings of considerable apprehension about what to say! On reflection I was puzzled by this because I considered myself to be a fairly sociable person, able to talk to my friends and to other people in new situations fairly readily. Nevertheless I felt very bemused by my feelings and awkward when sitting down in proximity to patients. I recall feeling unclear as to what to say, not knowing how to respond if asked questions for which I did not know the answer, wanting to be helpful but not wanting to appear too foolish.

My memories are a mixture of standing at the edge of the bed and not knowing whether to sit down, but feeling awkward perched on the edge. So I was hovering on the arm of the chair beside the bed. I looked as if I was about to spring off into some action which was terribly important. These were my defences used in order to appear more confident in what I was doing. Gradually, as I got to know the patients as individuals I began to feel more confident, I was able to relax as I worked, and lost most of the anxieties when I felt more a part of the health team.

On reflection these feelings were repeated at the beginning of all my placements. It took me between one and two weeks, depending on the area, to really settle.'

Elizabeth's honest account of her early experiences clearly illustrates the anxieties and lack of confidence common to the majority of staff at first. For some staff it can feel like entering an arena. It is clear how the carer's need to feel immediately able to care for patients may lead to anxious feelings of being 'de-skilled'.

It is therefore important that the carer has a clear understanding of what 'interpersonal skills' actually are. One of the difficulties for most health care workers is that the term 'interpersonal skills' is very ill-defined. A search through the current available literature does not help. 'Interpersonal skills' is an umbrella term used synonymously to mean communication skills, counselling skills, or any manner of skill involving some form of interaction, one to one or one to group (Fig. 1.2). Kagan (1985) defines interpersonal skills:

> 'As those aspects of both communication and social skills that are concerned with direct person to person contact'.

(Kagan, 1985)

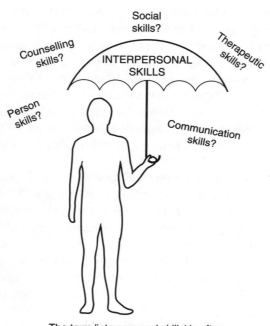

The term 'interpersonal skills' is often used synonymously with other terms.

**Fig. 1.2**   Interpersonal skills.

However, this needs to be focused more closely on the process of 'person-to-person' elements of interaction. Then it will be possible to identify more clearly behaviour which can be changed. For example, what are the desirable behaviours? How is 'person-to-person' communication improved? Is a 'communication skill' the same as an 'interpersonal skill?'

Although good interpersonal skills are generally accepted as essential and valuable for good patient care, there is increasing evidence which suggests that health workers do not communicate very well with patients, colleagues or other health professionals (Ashworth, 1980; Faulkner, 1980; MacLeod-Clark, 1985). Gijbels (1993) discusses possible reasons why interpersonal skills are not carried out very effectively by nurses. For example, he applies the findings of authors such as Hunt (1981) and Greenwood (1984) who explore how nurses use and implement research findings. He argues that nurses do not use interpersonal skills because:

- They do not fully understand the importance of using these skills.
- They do not believe in them, or they are not given incentives to implement them in practice, and therefore do not perceive them as relevant.

These explanations could almost certainly be applied to other health workers in this context. Gijbels (1993) also argues that effective communication and good interpersonal skills may not *really* be desired by health organisations. Quoting Graham (1981), he argues that power and control are often maintained by leaving 'things fuzzy'. Articulate and assertive communicators may be a nuisance, making demands which the organisation cannot meet. He suggests that in British culture particularly, the virtue 'silence is golden', serves as a subtle resistance to effective communication. He concludes that it is essential for the future that attention is given to clear theoretical frameworks for interpersonal skills teaching.

## Starting with 'self'

The practice of health care is a very stressful occupation. It is often for this reason that many interpersonal textbooks discuss the importance of 'self-awareness'. This is the skill of being personally alert to what one actually feels and responding in an honest way.

Health carers will often experience feelings that are confusing and disturbing. Such feelings are often stirred up in response to having to deal with a wide variety of human suffering; this can include dealing with individuals in pain, or with those who are totally dependent on the health setting for their survival. These emotions are often accompanied by fear and feelings of guilt which spring from a lack of confidence in how to be helpful or effective. Thus there is a mixture of fear and inadequacy and a resultant lack of self-confidence.

A fairly graphic example of these ambivalent and confusing feelings is given by Elizabeth at the beginning of this chapter. At first she describes the sensation of 'not knowing the ground rules and wanting desperately to blend in with the others in the caring team'. Certainly, in the early days of practice, the health worker may experience feelings which fluctuate between incompetence and insecurity, but which give way eventually to a growing sense of being able to attend to patients' needs. It is important for the health worker to understand these initial feelings, as a common experience. Carers must feel able to discuss their experiences with a trusted colleague or a 'mentor'. For many carers this is the first encounter with serious illness or death.

It is important to understand that powerful social and cultural rules exist in each health setting, whether a ward, clinic or community placement. Such rules have a very powerful effect upon the behaviour of the carer. For example, there are ground rules which have to be learnt when first entering the heath care field. Many of these 'rules' are often unconscious or implicit, with their origins in the past and the reasons for them now forgotten. This has been highlighted in the work of Isabel Menzies-Lyth (1988).

Menzies-Lyth attempted to understand the defences and strategies that nurses use in order to cope with the day-to-day anxieties of their work. In her study she applied 'psychodynamic theory' (described later in Chapter 2) in an attempt to understand the subtle 'rules' within nursing practice. This approach provides an understanding of the processes which ultimately affect the way nurses interact with one another and with patients. These processes also provide ways of dealing with the anxiety created by tense situations in the working environment. In her study, Menzies-Lyth argues that nurses are affected by the full weight of patients' anxieties. The mechanisms which are set up are often unconscious; that is, they are not deliberately constructed, but nevertheless occur as a way of helping to prevent nurses becoming too close or too intimate with patients as 'individuals'. Thus they are an unconscious form of protection.

For example, one method is the 'splitting up' of the nurse–patient relationship through task assignment, so that rather than allocating care to individual patients, work is broken up into the allocation of jobs or tasks. In this process, the patient's individuality becomes minimised by 'procedures'. While task assignment is generally criticised by nurses, this method of care management is still to be found.

From her observations, Menzies-Lyth comments that a particular culture, 'with its own language', exists in health care. Abbreviations such as 'temps' or 'obs' help to provide a code or 'language' which is only understood within the medical team. This has the effect of creating distance between staff and patient.

Another example of the development of 'defences' that create barriers, is the use of uniforms. Uniforms create uniformity; they help to create a conformity and homogenise attitudes. This leads to what Holloway and Penson (1987) describe as 'a collective consciousness' which the wearing of uniforms enhances. It is part of an unconscious system of control, a symbol of authority which enhances the uniformity of attitudes and behaviour (Wondrak, 1989).

Menzies-Lyth suggested that the relaxation of all these various strategies would need careful consideration. Rituals and uniforms have an important function in helping health carers deal with the traumas and anxieties that are part of their work. Therefore it is not surprising that students often find it difficult to implement what they may be taught about interpersonal skills. If the structures that exist in the institution run contrary to more open and clear interpersonal contact, carers will find themselves split between institutional conventions and genuine and honest communication. Traditional ways of teaching interpersonal skills may fail to provide the carer with the appropriate skills to make sense of these experiences.

Morse (1991), for example, argues that there is still a gap in the preparation of health workers to deal with these experiences and that in health care, communication classes are still teaching 'knee-jerk' responses – if the patient feels X then the practitioner says or does Y. This feels very artificial to the carer. An example of this may be in Elizabeth's account of feeling puzzled by her anxiety about talking to patients when instructed to do so by her senior. Often there is an expectation that the carer's new role as a professional carer will get in the way of simply listening to what the patient is saying, or of interacting in a natural way. When this does occur, the carer may feel inadequate and unsure of her role. It is for this reason that thinking more openly about personal feelings relating to what is experienced in the health care setting is so important; to consider and realise the confusing emotions that are likely to occur and to accept this as a natural part of the learning process.

In order to overcome some of these inherited cultural impediments to open communication, it is necessary to have a clear idea of the underlying theoretical frameworks and how these are linked to skills. These are considered in the next chapter.

# References

Ashworth, P. (1980) *Care of Communication: An Investigation into Problems of Communication Between Patients and Nurses in Intensive Therapy Units.* Royal College of Nursing, London.

Dryden, W. (1984) *Handbook of Individual Therapy in Britain Today.* Harper & Row, London.

Faulkner, A. (1980) *The student nurses' role in giving information to patients.* M. Litt. thesis, Aberdeen University.

Fulford, K.W.M., Ersser, S. and Hope, T. (1996) *Essential Practice in Patient-Centred Care.* Blackwell Science, Oxford.

Gijbels, H. (1993) Interpersonal skills training in nurse education: some theoretical and curricular considerations. *Nurse Education Today* **13**, 458–65.

Graham, R.J. (1981) Understanding the benefits of poor communication. *Interface,* **II**, 80–82.

Greenwood, J. (1984) Nursing research: a position paper. *Journal of Advanced Nursing* **9**, 77–82.

Holloway, I. and Penson, J. (1987) Nurse education as social control. *Nurse Education Today* **7**(5), 235–42.

Hunt, J. (1981) Indicators for nursing practice: the use of research findings. *Journal of Advanced Nursing* **6**, 189–94.

Kagan, C.M. (1985) (ed.) *Interpersonal Skills in Nursing: Research and Applications.* Chapman and Hall, London.

MacLeod-Clark, J. (1985) *Nurse-patient verbal interaction.* PhD thesis, University of London.

Menzies-Lyth, I. (1988) *Defence Systems as Control Against Anxiety.* Tavistock, London.

Morse, J.M. and Johnson, J.L. (1991) *The Illness Experience.* Sage Publications, California, USA.

Wondrak, R.F. (1989) Uniform actions. *Nursing Times* May 31, **85**, No. 22, 58–59.

# Further reading

Sundeen, S.J., Stuart, G.W., Rankin, E.A.D. and Cohen, S.A. (1994) *Nurse–Client Interaction,* 5th edn, Mosby, Chicago, USA.

# Chapter 2
# Theoretical Approaches

The three frameworks described in this chapter have had a significant influence on the understanding of human behaviour. Consequently, they also provide different perspectives on how to engage in an inter-personal way with others. Awareness of these approaches allows the health professional to act in a more therapeutic way with people. Over the many years since they were first described as theories that explain human behaviour, they have each become integrated into several frameworks used by health workers. This chapter will revisit each theory in detail, as it is a central argument of this book that the three approaches are *key* ideas in the development of effective interpersonal skills. For example, research suggests that being aware of the underlying theoretical position when interacting with patients is more effective than a 'haphazard' approach (Dryden, 1986).

The three approaches covered are:

- psychodynamic
- behavioural
- person-centred.

The approaches are often included in psychological texts, but are seldom included in the general literature, as *frameworks for exploring interactions* between the practitioner and the patient.

## The psychodynamic approach

The work of Sigmund Freud sets up a variety of reactions, many of them negative. This is unfortunate, given the contribution made by his work.

Many of the reactions are often misconceived and gleaned from assorted sources, many of which are inaccurate.

The term 'psychodynamic' is used because it refers to the belief that unconscious mental activity influences behaviour. Freud developed this theory as a result of his clinical observations, noting that factors often outside conscious attention influence action. Therefore 'psychodynamic' refers to the *process* of internal mental life and 'psychoanalysis' refers to the *method* of analysing these unconscious elements and exploring the inherent meaning for the individual.

The psychodynamic methods described in this book, while related to the ideas put forward by Freud, are not about psychoanalytical method. This distinction is important.

Freud's major contribution to our understanding of the mind, was his work on 'unconscious' mental life. Prior to Freud, people were viewed as being rational human beings who's intellects made them free to choose courses of action and behaviour which suited them best. Reason was the main determinant of how a person behaved and this concept, called 'rationalism' was the predominant view. A person was free to choose. The choices were 'weighed' up by the individual, who then made a decision based upon the best available information.

Philosophers in the late seventeenth and eighteenth centuries such as Descartes, Hobbes, Locke and Hume took a mechanistic view of behaviour. They suggested that some human actions did arise from forces which came from within the person and over which there is no control; for example, Hobbes argued that we behave in such a way as to achieve pleasure and avoid pain.

Freud, as well as being qualified in medicine, specialising in human physiology, was passionately interested in philosophy and made many important observations of human behaviour. He is often credited with developing one of the first comprehensive theories of the human mind. His basic assertions were that hidden below the surface of human consciousness, outside the range of an ordinary person's awareness, ideas and beliefs percolate and lie hidden from everyday awareness. Every event experienced by an individual from the time of their birth, or even before birth, has an effect. Although outside of immediate awareness, these experiences shape how a person behaves and may determine decision-making in later life. This is why this psychological approach is referred to as *psychodynamic psychology*.

The resistance to this explanation of human behaviour is understandable. No one likes to admit that choices are affected by anything other than conscious decision-making. An example may be seen in the underlying motivation for a career in the caring professions. There are several possible explanations. First, it may be that, along with a strong sense of public duty and a genuine desire to care for others, there is also a need to protect, in an unconscious way, the 'needy' parts of the self. This is an uncomfortable possibility for most people, who on the whole like to feel that they are in total control of what they think and how they behave. However, such an explanation may raise important awareness of behaviour which for some can assist interactions with others, raising consciousness of personal defences. During times of crisis such unconscious or *repressed* fears or feelings can suddenly come to the surface. For patients this is often when faced with illness and subsequent hospital care.

The concept of unconscious motivation and behaviour has met with resistance and has been rejected for being non-scientific (Webster, 1996). There are, however, three major areas of evidence of unconscious motives in human behaviour. These are:

- dreams
- slips and errors in everyday life
- symptoms that are sometimes expressed in our own behaviour.

Dreams are a complex phenomenon and physiological research continues to attempt to understand the function of dreaming. From a psychodynamic view, dreams are considered to be rich sources of material which assist in the understanding of anxiety. The basic position is that while asleep, the person is free of conscious control, which may 'censor' thinking. Dreams are confused free-ranging thoughts and can be helpful, alongside the patient's conscious consideration of feelings, in piecing together a more complex picture of mental life.

An example is a powerful dream experienced by the author's 10-year-old daughter. This occurred during an exchange visit to Australia. The first few months were stressful, settling into new schools and making new friends. The dream was of a large room divided by a thick glass wall. On one side of the glass was the school classroom at home. In this room were all her friends and a small native bird, the robin. On the other side of the glass wall was her current classroom in the new school. Native Australian parrots were perched on the shelves and several of her new friends were present. In the dream, she was unable to hear or speak to her friends through the glass because it was too thick, although she could see them all very clearly. The dream allowed a discussion of how much friends and familiar objects back at home were being missed and how the feeling of distance contributed to this. Discussing the dream at breakfast the next day allowed the feelings of loss and the feelings of frustration at 'not being able to speak to her friends' to be expressed.

So-called 'slips', or 'Freudian slips', occur as spontaneous disclosures of true feelings which seem to pop out from nowhere. Most people have experienced this phenomenon, which clearly indicates that thinking is taking place at a subconscious level. Symptoms expressed by patients can also provide evidence of thinking at this level. Some of these are discussed next.

## Basic concepts

Freud's model of the human mind (Fig. 2.1) consists of three key components:

- the *id*
- the *ego*
- the *superego*.

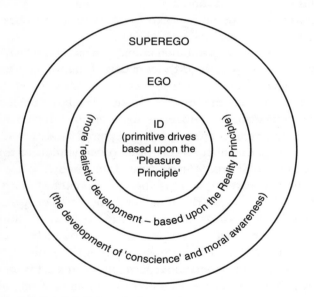

**Fig. 2.1**  Freud's model of the mind.

The infant personality consists mainly of what Freud called the *id*. This consists of two primitive drives necessary for survival. The id is based upon the *'pleasure principle'* and is motivated towards the satisfaction of basic desire.

As the infant grows, a much clearer definition of the world existing outside of itself develops. This is the beginning of the *ego*, a system of defences which enable the pressures of fulfilling the basic needs of the id to be kept in balance. The ego is based upon the *'reality principle'*. Freud argued that the ego is a part of the awareness which begins to develop as a response to 'external reality', the real restraints of life. The ego is the part of 'self' which polices the opposing drives of the id.

Later in life, nearing adolescence, a final and much more sophisticated 'layer' to the personality develops which Freud called the *superego*. Freud postulated that this was concerned with ideas of right and wrong and the development of *conscience*. For example if an individual feels very angry towards someone at work, the feeling may have to be suppressed if ventilation of anger is likely to be viewed badly by others. Thus the id, the source of basic primitive desire, has to be contained. A *rationalisation* takes place. This is mainly the ego 'considering the actions' of any outward show of aggression which may reflect badly. The angry feelings may then be stifled and suppressed. However, the internal frustrations remain and may 'leak out' later, to be taken out on a partner, or *displaced* onto other objects. The superego in this instance may form the basis of a 'higher' level of internal mediation of the conflict, and represent a more 'moral' view. Thus there may be some expunging of the feelings, through internal 'appeals' to conscience. The effect is to feel *guilt*.

In summary, the id is the source of primitive angry feelings, present even in those who find it hard to feel or express angry or hurtful feelings. The ego, is the more 'reasoning' part of personality, which attempts to contain the stronger feelings, according to what is perceived as acceptable behaviour at that time. The superego is a personal source of values and beliefs which have a governing function upon behaviour.

## Anxiety

The function of the ego is to mediate between the demands of the id and the superego. The id is concerned with instant gratification, the 'I want' part of self. The superego acts as the mature, 'adult-orientated' part of self. The ego functions as a 'buffer', reducing the tension that is created by the two demands.

Freud was concerned with describing psychological mechanisms and made an analogy with the 'homeostatic' mechanisms which occur within the human body. Such mechanisms maintain a balance, or equilibrium, within the body. Examples are the normal fluid balance or control of blood pressure. Similarly the mind can be considered as having developed mechanisms, which, as part of the personality, adjust the amount of anxiety or frustration experienced in life.

In this model, the individual strives to live peaceably in the world, balancing inner needs with reality. Conflict which builds up or cannot be contained, creates an anxious state. Anxiety can be defined as a state of painful internal tension associated with apprehension (Maddison *et al.*, 1971). Feeling anxious or tense is a fairly universal experience; however, it is very difficult to describe such feelings in words. Anxiety is perceived as an internal state of tension, conflict, apprehension, and 'butterflies in the stomach'. Often these feelings are associated with:

- restlessness
- insomnia
- physiological or physical symptoms such as headaches, stiffness, and gastric upsets
- physiological changes such as sweaty palms, rapid pulse and, in some circumstances, feelings of faintness and disability, or panic.

Anxiety acts as a 'warning of a state of threat', from which the individual needs to retreat, usually brought about by circumstances over which the individual has no control.

According to psychodynamic theory the origins of anxiety and frustration occur very early in life. Infants at a very early age realise that the demands of the id are unable to be satisfied straight away. The infant screams when hungry or for attention, which cannot always be met immediately. Thus the development of the 'reality principle' becomes the ego's emerging sense of what is possible and what is not! As this sense of reality grows, it is accompanied by a growing sense of *'self - identity'*. Self-identity refers here to a developing awareness of existing as an individual in a world full of objects or other people. For the infant, the mother or significant carer is soon viewed as being powerful, capable of taking away the unpleasant feelings, such as hunger. The degree of contentment that the infant feels depends upon the consistency of caring and love shown. The presence of a loving environment is necessary for the infant to develop personal confidence, self-esteem and to feel secure.

At this stage the infant is very dependent: when attention is withdrawn, or if it is lacking in the first place, then the infant's sense of security disappears and acute anxiety and helplessness is experienced. This situation is referred to as anxiety 'aroused by loss' (Bowlby, 1981). If the child receives adequate and continuous caring, he is more able to develop a sense of internal security and personal self-esteem. Where consistent care has been denied the child, he may grow into an adult who reacts adversely to stresses in later life.

At the beginning of Chapter 1, Elizabeth described feeling insecure when starting a new clinical placement. Everyday objects familiar to her provided security, as they conveyed a sense of familiarity. Thus when patients are admitted to hospital they may bring small items to display on their lockers. Photographs of family, friends or pets can help to reassure patients who have to spend longer periods of time away from their homes.

## Mental defence mechanisms

The mental defence mechanisms, or ego defence mechanisms as they are sometimes referred to, are the unconscious processes, employed to reduce or cope with internal anxiety. One way of attempting to understand these mechanisms is to draw an analogy with the physical defence mechanisms, such as the white blood cells (phagocytes) which tend to engulf invading bacteria. They are part of the natural protective defence for the body against infection. However if the individual is debilitated, or if the onslaught of bacterial attack is particularly vigorous, the immune system is unable to cope. Similarly the ego defence mechanisms help to protect against stress and anxiety in everyday life. This occurs as a mainly unconscious action: the mechanism 'clicks-in' automatically. All mechanisms except two are unconscious.

## Rationalisation and suppression

The two conscious mechanisms are:

- rationalisation
- suppression.

A good example of rationalisation is the typical smokers excuse: 'well I know it's dangerous to smoke but I may get knocked down crossing the road'. While rationalisations often contain an essence of truth, they are exaggerated and the individual is *consciously* aware of this. This mechanism is therefore employed in order to justify actions. Another example which the carer may recognise is that during some disappointment such as failing an examination, it is much easier to blame the examiner or 'wrong questions', than to admit personal failure.

Suppression is a consciously recognised process where the individual pushes an unpleasant or fearful memory, thought or feeling out of their mind. This is a type of *'motivated forgetting'* such as saying 'I don't want to think about it.'

The remaining mechanisms are all **unconscious** and these are now discussed.

## Sublimation

This is a common and healthy mechanism associated with reducing tension and anxiety. It is the process whereby all frustrations, conflicts, feelings or desires are **channelled** into socially acceptable forms. Often the tension is related to feelings of anger or aggression. Alternatively it may be concerned with sexual arousal or desire, particularly where this can not be immediately gratified. As sexual desire can only be satisfied within certain social situations, the demands of the id – the pleasure-seeking part of self – has to be contained. Sublimation is the channelling of these energies into socially acceptable activities, for example playing active sport or other physical activities which compensate such need.

According to Freud this mechanism is central to *catharsis* or release of energy, and thus forms one of the underlying theories of human motivation. Sublimation allows the more 'basic human drives' to be directed into more creative pursuits. It contributes extensively to the development of all creative activity, to the arts, and may even explain the underlying motivation to climb mountains. It is a 'safety valve' like the valve on a pressure cooker, which releases the energy when the pressure builds up inside. This idea gives some significance to internationally competitive sporting events, such as the Olympic Games. If it were not for these more healthy ways of discharging competitiveness, rivalries and jealousies that occur between nations might escalate and develop into war!

The next three mechanisms can be referred to as the 'three Rs' of unconscious defence.

## Repression

Repression is one of the first mechanisms described by Freud. When emotion is experienced as too threatening or troubling for the individual to deal with, the feelings can become deeply buried in the unconscious part of the mind. The mechanism is completely unconscious: once repressed there is no recollection of the disturbing thoughts. This mechanism allows us to live with the parts of ourselves we would rather not acknowledge. While it allows toleration of unpleasant thoughts by putting them 'out of mind' it can become unhealthy if it is used constantly as a way of blocking off feeling. An example of this mechanism is when we 'forget' that we owe somebody money, or completely forget a dental appointment. In more extreme situations, memories can be 'split off'. This is possible in very serious cases of shock, where the individual may have no recollection of events, or even forget parts of the past.

*Clinical example*

A clinical example is after a traumatic event, such as a car accident or a personal attack. Patients may recall only the events leading up to the incident, but have total amnesia for the actual episode. This process can be explained as a repression of those very painful disturbing events which enable the patient to 'switch off'. It is a protection against having to face the immediate events surrounding the trauma, giving space and time to digest what has happened. In events such as this, recall often returns; however, in more severe cases, repression may continue for a long time. When this happens, the first sign may be an associated anxiety, without awareness of what the reason may be, the origins being repressed long ago.

## Reaction formation

Reaction formation is best described as an unconscious, self-induced mechanism which attempts to change a strong emotion into its opposite.

*Clinical example*

After a long and tiring shift, Sarah arrived home feeling tired and completely worn out. After a hot bath, feet up, and looking forward to a relaxing meal and an evening in front of the television, the door bell rings. Looking out through the curtains, a colleague has turned up for the evening. Although a friend and usually very welcome, Sarah dreads this tonight, as all she wants to do is relax and watch TV! However, the friend has seen the curtains move and it is impossible for Sarah to pretend she is not in – a thought that did pass through her mind! With some resignation she opens the front door – but instead of saying how she really feels, Sarah greets her friend with an exaggerated welcome!

Sarah finds herself behaving in the opposite way, not conveying her true feelings, but working hard to convey the opposite.

In a similar situation many people would be able to feel assertive enough to express how they truly feel. However, a large number of people can not. This is especially true among health care workers!

A 'reaction formation' can be described as a statement of feeling or belief which is *opposite* to what is really felt. It is as though the individual says 'I do not desire something which is unacceptable: on the contrary I desire the very opposite' (Maddison *et al.*, 1971).

Reaction formation is often the opposite of personal characteristics or personality traits. For example an individual who is very authoritarian and who tries to portray the impression of being in control and 'in charge' may be reacting against internal feelings of low self-esteem and insecurity. Another example is someone who appears to be very cold, aloof and indifferent in their relationships with others. The message seems to be 'I do not need anyone else's love or attention'. However, this outward demeanour betrays an intense feeling of fear of other people and of intimate relationships. The fear is usually related to a fear of being rejected, or else a fear of becoming dependent upon someone else. Their reaction is a protection against getting hurt.

## Regression

Regression is a mechanism which literally means reverting back to an earlier stage of development, where behaviour becomes very childlike. Such behaviour increases during times of anxiety, fear or intense stress. It is a temporary denial of adult responsibility.

The process enables the person to have a space or 'time out' from the stressful situation and to 'let off steam'.

### Clinical example

In the health care context, the patient may assume a very dependent role, behaving in a very immature way or becoming very demanding. The institutional structure of health care often encourages such dependence, for example the use of uniforms and hierarchical relationships.

## Displacement

This is an important mental defence mechanism and one readily recognised by practitioners in clinical practice. Displacement enables the individual to reduce anxiety by displacing or transferring feelings, such as guilt or anger, on to another object.

### Clinical example

An example is where a carer feels anger towards a senior colleague. Rather than expressing this, the anger is contained until it can be more safely expressed. This usually occurs by directing the feelings towards inanimate objects, such as slamming doors, but may also be an innocent partner, who may end up totally nonplussed.

A more extreme situation can be seen in psychiatric practice, where anxiety is displaced on to a specific situation or object. This is a *phobic reaction*. An example is the condition *agoraphobia*, where an individual becomes frightened of situations involving being in crowded places or anywhere unfamiliar.

A specific skill that the carer is required to develop in such instances is to examine the situation for the presence of *'secondary gain'*. Secondary gain is where an unconscious advantage is achieved through development of the symptom. This often occurs despite the obvious discomfort and incapacity it creates for the person. In agoraphobia, for instance, incapacity becomes the focus of considerable attention. It is by the careful examination of secondary gain that clues about the underlying cause of the problem can usually be found. Often, this is linked to unfulfilled or unsatisfactory relationships in the person's life.

### Denial

This is a classic defence mechanism whereby unacceptable facts, beliefs or desires are totally removed from any acknowledgement of existence. It is a primitive mechanism which has its roots in early childhood development. A very young child will often believe that the world has 'disappeared' when he closes his eyes. Or the tired child, who despite visibly falling asleep will insist on 'not being tired!' – a complete denial of the reality.

In clinical disorders there is a process of *disowning* or refusing to acknowledge reality, because to do so would be painful or threatening. For instance denial is a mechanism often seen in people with drinking disorders, where there is a refusal to believe that there is a real problem.

*Clinical example*

An example occurs during the breaking of bad news. The person informed of a terminal disease, such as cancer, reacts with a period of disbelief and denial that it has really happened to them.

Maddison *et al.* (1971) give another example of a type of denial which is often displayed in patient behaviour, where the patient becomes very euphoric. In this particular instance the person becomes excessively and abnormally cheerful, in a way which is totally incongruent with the situation. Such an example is a mixture of both denial and reaction formation. (Reaction formation is described earlier in this chapter.)

Denial is a common ego defence against acceptance of painful truths and can be seen in the reactions to severe illness that many patients display.

| Mechanism | Description and function |
|---|---|
| Sublimation: | channelling of aggressive or other 'unacceptable' drives into socially acceptable pursuits. Serves to reduce aggressive or sexual tension. |
| Repression: | unconscious 'forgetting' of painful or traumatic events. Serves as a protection against emotional overload. |
| Reaction formation: | the unconscious reversion of strong emotion into the portrayal of the opposite expression. Serves to protect individual from being rejected by others. |
| Regression: | reverting to immature ways of behaving at times of stress. Serves to reduce tension. |
| Displacement: | transferring the real source of frustration onto objects that are perceived to be more safe. Serves to reduce anxiety, however often leads to avoidance of the true cause. |
| Denial: | the unconscious blocking of events that have a basis in reality. Serves to prevent acceptance of unacceptable truths. |

**Fig. 2.2**   Mental (ego) defence mechanisms.

*Summary*

In summary, there are a number of mental (ego) defence mechanisms (Fig. 2.2) which, according to Freud, are processes developed by the mind to enable the person to deal with day-to-day stress. Freud argued that his endeavour was to 'transform human misery into common everyday unhappiness'. He has often been criticised for having a very pessimistic view of human nature; later theorists propose a more positive view (Carl Jung, for example, split with Freud and developed his own psychodynamic view of the unconscious.)

The defence mechanisms function as 'homeostatic' processes, managing the reduction of anxiety. When stress is at such a level that the individual can not cope, or that the defence mechanisms are insufficient to be able to deal with the anxiety, the individual will be at risk of ill health.

This view of human interaction is controversial; however, it is possible to see how the processes described can cause the behaviour that is experienced by carers both within themselves and in their patients. This approach does offer an explanation for how people behave in times of stress or crisis.

# The behavioural approach

Behavioural theory may be described as an approach which focuses upon the way in which an individual repeats or learns behaviour, as a result of reward or reinforcement, and that such principles determine all or most of human behaviour.

## Classical conditioning

The earliest development of these ideas is associated with the work of Ivan Pavlov (1927) and the *conditioned reflex*. This is a form of associative learning often described as a *stimulus response* set of behaviours. Pavlov was studying autonomic reflexes, the part of the nervous system which operates in an automatic way. At the time of his discovery he was working on the salivary glands in dogs. The dogs would obviously salivate in response to food; however, he also noticed salivation occurring *before* the food was presented to the animal. This puzzled him.

Pavlov was a very methodical worker and always fed the dogs at the same time each day. This would coincide with a university bell that would ring to announce lunchtime. One day he was slightly late, and before any food could be brought in for the dogs, the bell rang, and he noticed the dogs salivating in response to the bell.

He went on to successfully teach dogs to salivate by various signals, such as pairing the ring of the bell or the flashing of a light with the reward of food (Fig. 2.3). This became known as *classical conditioning*. The significance of this discovery was that it was possible to learn to adapt natural 'innate' behaviour in both animals and humans, and condition the response to a new set of stimuli.

## Operant conditioning

Much of this theory was later developed by psychologists, notably by John Watson who has been described as the founder of behaviourism. However the work of Burrhus F. Skinner (1953) is more often associated with this approach to understanding human behaviour. Burrhus F. Skinner was born in 1904, in Pennsylvania USA. He was particularly interested in the science of behaviour and became an experimental scientist interested in searching for rational explanations for human behaviour.

Skinner went on to develop a variation to the conditioned response described by Pavlov. He observed that it was possible to encourage behaviour that did not depend upon the animals 'normal reflex' action, such as salivation. He demonstrated that behaviour not related to the normal range of behaviour associated with a specific animal, could be conditioned. He called the method *operant conditioning*, emphasising the fact that the behaviour 'operates' on the environment to generate the change in behaviour.

Both classical and operant conditioning rely upon regular reinforcement or the use of rewards and there are important rules governing how behaviour can be encouraged. If a reward does not immediately follow the behaviour that is required, the desired behaviour will not be repeated. Behaviourism emphasises the importance of rewards, and this is considered to be part of the normal process of human development. Thus praise from people important to us, love or attention, are important reward mechanisms.

Skinner also found that if rewards are continuous, that is if the reinforcement is continually supplied, the subject becomes disinterested and the conditioning fails. It appears that motivation or attention is lost; there is no need to act or perform the behaviour required because the reward is constant.

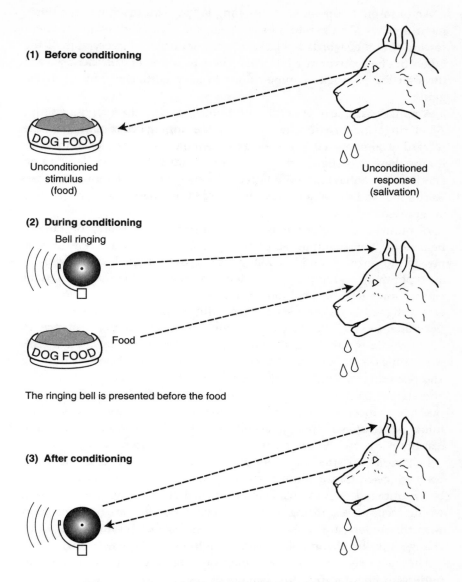

**(1) Before conditioning**

Unconditionied
stimulus
(food)

Unconditioned
response
(salivation)

**(2) During conditioning**

Bell ringing

Food

The ringing bell is presented before the food

**(3) After conditioning**

Ringing bell (conditioned stimulus) produces salivation as a response (this is now called a
*conditioned response*)

**Fig. 2.3**   Pavlov's conditioning experiment.

An example of operant conditioning is the 'fruit machine' in amusement arcades. The machine is so designed that it gives intermittent reward; in other words the jackpot does not occur at every spin of the wheel but happens at rare intervals. There is, however, sufficient reward through the payback of minor sums to keep sufficient interest in the game.

Another example of operant conditioning is when the telephone rings. A bell rings and an association between the ringing bell is made with the reward of someone talking. If every time the phone was picked up after it rang there was silence, the behaviour would not be rewarded and no conditioning behaviour would occur. Because we do not know who may be ringing, and some calls are more 'rewarding' than others, the process is repeated.

A number of experiments demonstrated conditioning of human behaviour. For example Verplanck (1955) demonstrated how it was possible to verbally condition a student in a psychology class. Unaware of an experiment taking place, a student was engaged in what he thought was an informal conversation with a tutor. However, the conversation was designed to follow a set pattern, with the intention of conditioning the student to include the words 'I think' or 'I believe' in a sentence; in other words to reinforce statements of opinion made by the student. Every time the student used those words the tutor would be very positive and responded with the words 'you are right' or 'I agree'. By doing this and stating the intentions beforehand, Verplanck demonstrated it was possible to increase the number of times the student used the words 'I think' or 'I believe', thereby establishing that it is possible to verbally condition a person to say particular words more often.

Behaviourism stresses the importance of learning and as such has been criticised for the mechanistic way in which certain behaviours can be encouraged or reinforced. Interpersonal skills using this approach would focus on rewarding the desired behaviour, and are not concerned with the underlying causes, or reasons for the behaviour that is to be changed. In this theory, all behaviour is the product of learning.

The next section will examine the **person-centred approach** to understanding interpersonal behaviour.

## 'Person-centred' approaches

The person-centred (or client-centred) approach is quite different from the psychodynamic or behavioural approaches which have been described so far in this chapter. This approach emphasises the central importance of the individual's belief about self, personal values and interests, and the importance of the way in which a person functions in the present. There is less of a focus upon childhood history, with more appraisal of the 'here and now'.

Two key individuals associated with these ideas and their translation into clinical practice are Abraham Maslow (1970) and Carl Rogers (1969, 1980). These writers belong to a school of psychology that became known as the *humanistic school*. The term person-centred is an adaptation of the humanistic approach used by Rogers (1969). This was a tradition that gained momentum in the late 1950s , largely as a reaction against the mechanistic explanations of human behaviour offered by the behavioural school. Person-centred theory is rooted in the principles of humanistic psychology, which is more concerned with understanding interpersonal interaction.

Person-centred is a very positive view of human behaviour and, as the name suggests, refers to the belief that the 'person' is central, with strengths, aspirations and conscious free will. There is an inherent belief that every person is capable of fulfilling personal ambitions and reaching their full potential.

## Development of person-centredness

Early in life the child starts to develop a view of 'self' which develops into a *self-concept*. Humanistic writers often make a distinction between self-concept and self. Nelson-Jones (1982) clarifies this distinction by suggesting that the 'self' should be regarded as the real or underlying part of the person, essentially trustworthy and striving towards realisation of full potential or *self-actualization*. Self-concept, however, develops over a lifetime and is affected by the attitudes of family, friends, care takers and significant others (Fig. 2.4).

It follows that the two views may become very different. The 'self' concept is a view that we have about ourselves in order to gain appreciation and satisfaction through recognition from others. The 'real self' is the more central core, which contain more truthful feelings. This gives a different view of human nature and can be contrasted with the discussion earlier in this chapter concerning Freud's view of the id and ego. Thus the humanist model, although recognising that people are influenced by their childhood, differs very much from the psychodynamic view, placing much more importance on the so-called 'here and now', on what is actually happening in the present rather than the past.

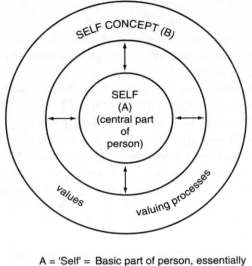

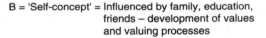

A = 'Self' = Basic part of person, essentially
trustworthy, striving towards full
potential

B = 'Self-concept' = Influenced by family, education,
friends – development of values
and valuing processes

**Fig. 2.4**   Person-centred model of development.

The self-concept gradually becomes organised as sets of values or valuing processes. These soon start to come into conflict with parents or other significant caretakers. According to this view, conflict arises between the self-concept and the impositions created by the external world. Also, Rogers was one of the first to recognise the importance of the concept of *unconditional positive regard*, being central and very different to other approaches.

Unconditional positive regard is the process of valuing another person in a positive way, demonstrating love and concern no matter how he behaves. In developmental terms, behaviour that is unacceptable is made clear so that the child learns the difference between right and wrong; however the fundamental interpersonal communication is that the child is loved and cared for, even when being told off. Rogers (1969), argued that this was a key device, defined as the regard for other people without judgement, and expressed through the development of under-standing. He suggested that this was crucial for the development of a healthy self-concept and self-confidence.

## *Empathy*

Empathy is an important concept in the formation of relationships. It is described as the capacity to 'put oneself into the other person's position' in order to appreciate how they may be feeling. In reality this is a very difficult task, as clearly some patients' circumstances will be beyond the carer's ability to fully appreciate. A more workable definition of the concept is the ability to be able to understand the context from which another person is operating; for example, by trying to imagine the situation of a patient and attempting to understand his feelings. This skill requires attentive listening and attention to the detail in the patient's descriptions of his experience.

## *Hierarchy of needs*

Maslow was a leader in the development of humanistic psychology. He argued that specific human needs lead to internal drives towards satisfying them. He proposed a *hierarchy of needs* (Fig. 2.5). Maslow argued that human motivations arise from basic biological needs present at birth, gradually increasing in complexity. The needs at one level have to be at least partially satisfied before the needs of the next level motivate a change of behaviour. So for example when food and water are the primary need, the other needs are not as important to an individual. In this approach, only when the satisfaction of basic needs has been satisfied does energy for higher needs occur.

For Maslow, the final goal, at the top of the ladder, is self-actualisation – the search for self-fulfilment or realisation of self-potential. Maslow argued that very few individuals actually achieve this state. Most continue to strive towards self-actualising.

The person-centred approach begins with the assumption that all individuals are basically trustworthy and that 'trust' arises from a belief that all organisms possess an underlying drive towards self-fulfilment. This is a very different view of human nature, to the more pessimistic psychodynamic view.

In recent years the person-centred approach has been criticised for disregarding the darker side of human nature. Theological critics particularly, have condemned it for naïvety and absence of any negative view that might equate to 'evil behaviour' in the world. The person-centred response would be that 'evil' itself does not exist as a concept. The humanistic view of human nature would suggest that conditions in

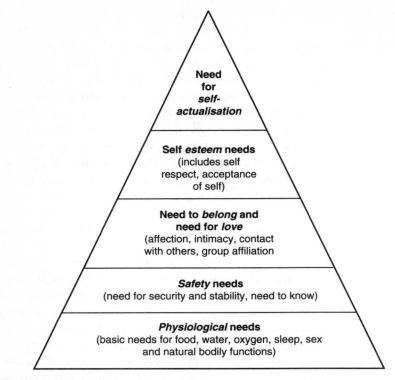

**Fig. 2.5**   Maslow's hierarchy of needs.

life create the behaviour, and that individuals are born innocent. This is a clearly different view again to psychodynamic theory which suggests a primitive centre of human personality – the pleasure-seeking id.

The person-centred tradition is that the individual *can* take responsibility for personal behaviour, possessing an inherent capacity to reorientate psychological positions from those of maladjustment to a state of psychological health. Such capabilities, however, are only present when the individual learns to become free of defensive behaviour, is more open to others, and learns more trustworthy ways (Reynolds and Cormack, 1990).

## Specific person-centred skills

According to Rogers (1969), important strategies are necessary to encourage sufficient growth. These are described as:

- warmth
- empathy
- genuineness

Empathy has been described earlier, as attempting to imagine how the person may be feeling, by thinking about their circumstances and listening carefully to descriptions of events.

Warmth or respect is a prerequisite to enabling a relationship to grow. It means being interested in the person as an *individual*, rather than a person with a disease. Sometimes this is very difficult to do in practice, because of various pressures at work, or because we simply find it difficult to like someone. Unconditional positive regard appears to be a sound theoretical idea, which is often difficult to realise; in practice all health workers will have their own prejudices and dislikes. However, it is good practice to try and understand, and respect another position. Moreover this is a fundamental responsibility of professional action. It is also important to indicate that where, in practice, this is very difficult, possibly for very good reasons, the alternative is to understand what is happening in the relationship – to put some 'boundary' around what the problem may be, and discuss it with a friend, colleague or mentor. This is what taking responsibility means in this context, rather than avoidance. Rogers believed that it is important for health professionals to be honest, recognise personal limitations, and confront them openly.

Genuineness is similar to being trusting and open; that is, avoiding pretence, without being defensive, authoritarian or manipulative. There is often a difficulty here for many carers, which is worth illustrating. Early in clinical experience the practitioner may find herself subjected to patients asking very searching and difficult questions. An example is where the carer may know that a patient has a terminal illness and is unsure what to say or how to respond in an honest way. Where this happens there is a dilemma. The practitioner knows that being honest and genuine is an important personal and professional quality, and yet confronted with the real-life situation of a desperate person turning to her and seeking a truthful answer, it may be very difficult. This is a dilemma faced by most practitioners, however it is likely to be the junior who is often working closest to the patient. The carer must be clear about the agreed policy of care. Health professionals may fudge the issue. They feel, perhaps naturally, inexperienced, unable to answer fully, and refer back to the person in charge.

Referring back is often the best solution when in doubt. However, clear communication is assisted by the way in which patient care is organised. This can be facilitated by not losing sight of the importance of trying to understand how the patient may be feeling and what questions they may ask.

## Conclusions

The three approaches described in this chapter set the scene for the discussion in the following chapters. While each approach offers a unique perspective on human interactive behaviour, each is not capable of discriminating, or giving sufficient explanation for the full range of human activity that the practitioner will experience. Often it may seem that behaviour can be understood by using parts of all three approaches to explain certain occurrences. This is to use an *eclectic approach*; in other words there may be several explanations to understand just one particular pattern of behaviour. Psychologists are not suggesting they have the answers for explaining all human behaviour.

The interpersonally skilled practitioner is the one who is aware of what theoretical approach, or approaches, influences the way they work with patients. There is evidence (Dryden, 1986) that this has been shown to be more therapeutically effective. A working knowledge of the above theories supplies the grounding for developing skilled interventions with patients. However, skilled interpersonal behaviour has also to begin with the carer being open enough to look critically at how she relates to others, being mindful of patterns of defensive behaviour.

## References

Bowlby, J. (1981) *Attachment and Loss*, Vol. 3. Penguin, Middlesex.
Dryden, W. (1986) *Individual Therapy in Britain*. Harper & Row, London.
Maddison, D., Day, P. and Leadbeater, B. (1971) *Psychiatric Nursing*. Churchill Livingstone, Edinburgh.
Maslow, A.H. (1970) *Motivation and Personality*. Harper & Row, New York.
Nelson-Jones, R. (1982) *The Theory and Practice of Counselling Psychology*. Cassell, London.
Pavlov, I.P. (1927) *Lectures on Conditioned Reflexes*. Liveright, New York.
Reynolds, W. and Cormack, D. (1990) *Psychiatric and Mental Health Nursing; Theory and Practice*. Chapman and Hall, London.
Rogers, C.R. (1969) *Freedom to Learn*. Charles E. Merrill, Columbus, Ohio.
Rogers, C.R. (1980) *A Way of Being*. Houghton Mifflin, Boston.
Skinner, B.F. (1953) *Science and Human Behaviour*. Macmillan, New York.

Verplanck, W.S. (1955) The control of the content of conversation: reinforcement of statements of opinion. *Journal of Abnormal and Social Psychology* **51**, 668–76.
Webster, R. (1996) *Why Freud was Wrong*. Harper Collins, London.

## Further reading

Freud, S. (1975) *The Psycopathology of Everyday Life: 5*. Penguin Books, Middlesex.
Freud, S. (1962, reprinted 1987) *Two Short Accounts of Psychoanalysis*. Pelican Books, Middlesex.
Skinner, B.F. (1974) *About Behaviourism*. Knopf, New York.

# Chapter 3
# Approaches to the Care of the Child

*Richard's account*

'I was really looking forward to my "children's placement"; most of my friends had worked there and I had a good idea of what to expect. Despite this, I remained frightened of what it would actually be like in practice. Some of the stories I had heard made me wonder how I would deal with the situations. Like a friend who was nursing a dying child, and another who had to look after a toddler who had sustained severe fractures in a fall, and was in considerable pain. I wondered how I would react, how I would cope emotionally, when the patient was a child and did not really understand what was happening. These were thus my first thoughts as I walked into ward 2 of the local children's hospital, a mixed-sex ward. Ages ranged from about 4 years to 12 years, although there was a 16-year-old who was receiving continuous chemotherapy and had been a patient there for the past four years.

I remember the 'atmosphere' seemed much more relaxed than my previous adult placements and the ward was much more colourful, and decorated with characters from Disney films. It felt, at least at first, a bit like entering a surreal theme park: a foreground of strange trolleys and instruments, with a brightly coloured background of posters, toys and teddies with bandaged limbs.

While looking forward to working in a new area, I always dread the first week of any new clinical placement. I have never found an easy way of dealing with not knowing anything and feeling totally inadequate. However, wanting to be "useful", learning the routines and concentrating on the people I would be caring for was the way I had always dealt with settling into any new area.

One of the first things to strike me was that I needed to develop new skills in communication. While I have a younger brother and sister, my experience of addressing the questions that were thrown at me, seemed inappropriate. For example I was asked in a very direct way "Why I had such a big nose . . . what I was going to do with the urine I collected from the bag" (whilst emptying and changing one), and if I was "going to throw it away", and if so "why was I bothering to collect it anyway!". Thus my previously honed nursing skills had not prepared me sufficiently for knowing how to respond in the most appropriate way. I knew that the essence of good communication was to be "genuine" and honest, but most of these kids were very curious about what was happening around them, and furthermore confronted me about it directly. Adults, it seemed to me, did not ask such awkward questions, although I suspected they would have liked to!

I was soon able to develop the skill of explaining what I was doing and for what reasons, in a more open way that was not too technical and, even more important, not condescending or patronising. I recall a particularly embarrassing moment when during an aspiration of a naso-gastric tube in a ten-year-old who asked me questions, I inadvertently slipped into "simplified language". I therefore referred to the "wind-pipe" and the "food pipe", in my hearty attempt to explain the complexities of testing that the tube was in the stomach . "Oh", he replied "you mean the trachea and oesophagus!". Then he described the anatomy and physiology of the upper thorax, explaining that he had *The Human Body* on CD-Rom! Needless to say I learnt an important lesson about treating children (and adults) with much more respect, and checking out with them first what they knew!

I did find nursing children to be very different from the other forms of nursing I had undertaken before. For instance, it was much more orientated towards the family. Even though all effective nursing care must by its nature involve the family of the patient, here it seemed to be a much more clear and direct involvement. One of my earliest memories of working on ward 2, was having to teach an eight-year-old how to give his own insulin injections. He was a very courageous lad; however, when it came to actually injecting himself he became tearful and asked me to do it. I knew that success in this endeavour would only mean allowing him to be able to carry out the whole procedure for himself. Thus I had to push him and be firm. This was a totally new experience for me and one which I found very difficult to carry out. This was particularly so when I also had to have his parents with him in order to teach them how to perform the task. At one point I recall all three were crying and I had to decide whether to pause or continue to see through what I was doing. I decided I had to carry on encouraging the patient to inject himself. Eventually, however, it all came together, and the patient and his parents became very adept at calculating doses, drawing up the syringe, and injecting the insulin.

For a while I also felt that I had very little to do. Most of the parents were being encouraged to give the care, and I felt confused about what I was supposed to be doing.

Another key difference is the patients themselves. I soon grew to like their directness and the brave ways in which they coped with sometimes very sad and painful conditions. I never really got to the point of accepting the death of a young child; however I found working and caring for these children a very satisfying and important nursing role'.

Richard's account raises a number of issues which many health workers new to this area of care experience. There is much more emphasis on allowing the parents, or significant relatives, to actually carry out much of the day-to-day care. As Richard discloses, this can occasionally create some uncertainty about the role at first, until the health worker feels more confident about how to assist both parent and child.

Working with children is a very challenging area of health care practice. Often the carer has to work with children who are undergoing frightening experiences, pain and discomfort, and at this time the significance of the relationship becomes the only effective way of trying to understand the communication that is attempted by the child. For example, when nursing a baby or very young children the importance of developing empathetic understanding becomes crucial. The child has a greater potential for misunderstanding, and the uncertainty created through fantasies the child may have about a procedure or intervention can increase the anxiety (Broome, 1986, 1990).

In a review of the literature related to caring for children, Brennan (1994) cites a number of studies that support the finding that the main fear of the child in hospital is a fear of 'bodily distortion' or of mutilation. Given the influence of television and the children's programmes that focus upon space age technologies and the often vivid portrayal of the destructive power of machines, it is not difficult to comprehend a child's fear of radiographic and other 'high tech' equipment that health workers take for granted. The author can still recall the vivid fear of a portable X-ray machine during a period of hospitalisation at the age of ten years. This machine looked like the 'Daleks' – robot machines from the children's television programme *Dr Who* that had a passion for 'exterminating' people! Such childhood fears can cause great anxiety.

Children's apprehension about procedures is often linked to family notions of illness and hospitalisation, usually communicated by a parent whose experiences of childhood illness were unhappy but are also now well out of date. Perrin and Gerrity (1981) argue that childhood fears about what will happen to them is also a function of the awareness they have of their own bodily functions. Children may also have a view of hospitals as unpleasant places where 'punishment' is carried out. This feeling may be linked to early feelings of guilt, or the result of some misdeed. Piaget (1977), the Swiss psychologist, referred to this tendency in some children as 'immanent justice'. Exploring childhood perceptions and developmental views held by children at different ages, helps the health staff to identify better with the feelings the child has about their condition.

The ability to be able to identify with the patient is, of course, one of the basic skills of all nursing care (Benner and Tanner, 1987). However, it is particularly difficult – a skill that is often the result of studied observation. For example, Rayner (1993) highlights the differences that appear in an infant's facial expression over the span of just a few months, which makes understanding them a difficult process. Staff may have to rely on the parents for assistance in interpretation.

'A baby moves in a cycle between sleep, arousal and distress; if disturbed in this he becomes distressed ... these three stages involve definable differences in the activity of the nervous system of adults as well as children. These are important to recognise when considering any sort of stress, anxiety, anger, defence and aggression.'

Rayner, 1993, p. 30)

Even the most inexperienced nurse will recognise that infants communicate through either crying, smiling or laughing. Considerable research has, and continues to be, undertaken to understand how babies and infants communicate and how best to care for children. Health staff can benefit by being more critically aware and selective of appropriate interventions. Brennan (1994) argues that caring for the child has a 'double challenge' – to care for the needs of the child and parents during a medical procedure and also to ensure that the procedure is performed effectively and professionally. Many parents will be able to carry out the procedures with the staff teaching and helping them.

Wolff (1969) has found that there are different patterns of crying. These consist of the infant's 'normal' rhythmic crying, and then the crying associated with anger, pain, discomfort or frustration. Crying is clearly an important way of attempting to understand the baby's experience. Usually the mother will learn to differentiate between the varying forms of crying, smiling and laughing in her own child. The health carer has to develop these skills through close observation and attention to how each infant responds.

There are clearly challenges for those working with the very ill child. This is a concern of many carers who commence a career working with children and mentioned by Richard in his account at the beginning of this chapter. For example, there is the difficulty of providing stimulation to the child who is being cared for surrounded by very delicate measuring instruments where movement is limited. The appearance of the child, fragile and in the midst of such sophisticated apparatus is itself a significant contributory factor to the stress that parents of the child also have to face (Goldson, 1992). The focus on the technology and need to survey the equipment can mean that fundamental interactions, such as touching or talking to the child, may at times be overlooked (D'Apolito, 1991).

Saunders (1994) has reviewed some of the research relating to the neonatal intensive care unit (NICU), and found studies that have highlighted how the deleterious effects of the 'sights and sounds of the NICU can be overwhelming to both infants and children alike'. There is an obvious barrier to the development of the relationship between adult and child. The hum of the equipment, gasps of the ventilators, bright overhead lights and general hyperactivity often associated with the unit can create 'overstimulation' and agitation in the child. A solution that has been gathering some momentum with carers is the playing of soft music or replaying the mother's voice as an antidote to the adverse environmental sounds (Stanley and Moore, 1995).

The development of the child and the common experiences of being cared for in health care contexts will now be reviewed. The three approaches introduced in the last chapter will be applied, focusing on the interpersonal relationship.

# The psychodynamic perspective

Early psychodynamic approaches consider the stages of early infant development as consisting of several *psychosexual stages* (Fig. 3.1, Freud, 1905). Babies develop through a number of developmental phases. The first stage is the 'oral stage'.

| Stage | Age: years | Characteristics |
|-------|-----------|-----------------|
| Oral | 0–1 | Exploration of sensations through mouth, sucking – instant gratification is sought. |
| Anal | 2–3 | Awareness of bodily functions – 'potty'-training phase. |
| Phallic | 4–5 | Preoccupation with genital area, awareness of differences between 'male' and 'female' physically. |

**Fig. 3.1**   Freud's psychosexual stages.

### *The oral stage (age 0–1 year)*

In this stage the child is primarily motivated to explore the sensations through the mouth, receiving gratification through sucking. Anything that is possible to be put into the mouth is directed there! Freud based this idea on his theory of personality development where he argued that the infant is primarily motivated by the drives of the id or pleasure-seeking principle, striving for instant gratification of innate desires for food and pleasure (see Chapter 2).

The psychological basis of the behaviour is to reduce anxiety present in the child's experience of the world, through the relief brought about from the pleasure of taking objects into the mouth. According to this theory, it is possible for an individual to become stuck or 'fixated' at this stage. An example in adulthood would be compulsive eating, smoking or nail biting. These behaviours increase during moments of tension or anxiety.

From a psychodynamic viewpoint, eating disorders in younger childhood, such as obsessive fastidiousness regarding food, or actual anorexia nervosa, may be linked to attempts by the child to reduce anxiety by controlling behaviour. Sudden change, illness or fear of loss, are instances where the child may react by attempting to manipulate and control eating behaviour. It is crucially important to emphasise that the child engages in this activity in an unconscious way. This behaviour has a hidden 'secondary gain' of achieving the adult's attention in a way that may be impossible for the child to express in any other way. It is not carried out in a premeditated, or calculated way.

For the health worker, important interpersonal skills to apply in such a situation would involve not confronting the child about the behaviour at this stage. Stepping back, reflecting on the 'total situation', allows more information to be assessed. The child can be offered understanding and reassurance. All clinical staff need to be informed about the child's behaviour and a consistent approach adopted. If the behaviour persists then it may become necessary to refer on to a child clinical psychologist for assessment. Essential skills would begin with attempting to understand how the child perceives the threat and what is creating the anxiety. Open-ended comments rather than direct questioning may be more effective, for example discussing how natural it is for many children to be frightened and anxious about coming into hospital, raising the issue in a general rather than directly challenging way.

## The anal stage (2–3 years)

This next stage is referred to as the 'anal stage'. This where the infant becomes more aware of their bodily functions and explores the pleasures (and power to be gained) from bowel movements! Normally, children learn through toilet training and eventually move successfully through this stage. According to Freud, late problems associated with this phase of development can be obsessive behaviours, particularly related to cleanliness and overconcern for neatness and order. For some children, deliberately creating messes, and in some more serious cases deliberately soiling the bed or walls, can be viewed as angry attempts to redress power and helplessness, or as an 'attack' on the adult. When children are worried or anxious there may be temporary bed-wetting or 'accidents'. Where this occurs it is very important to assess what may be going on, as such behaviour may be due to a variety of causes, both physiological and psychological. Physically, it may be due for example to pain, effects of medication, or fatigue. Psychologically it may be fear, anger at being in hospital or with parents for 'leaving them there', anxiety or a communication for help, in a small child who is bewildered.

Psychodynamically, there may be symbolic associations. Rayner (1993) points out that for a small child there may be a frightening equation between faeces and 'dead things'. He points out that after death, animals smell very much like faeces and this connection is very quickly picked up by the child, who associates them as being much alike. Thus in the imagination of the child, the anxiety about being in hospital may exaggerate the association and fears about annihilation (Rayner, 1993).

What may be more likely however is greater concern about

performing toilet activity. Depending on the age of the child there are likely to be complex fantasies about toilet functions, which are products of that child's toilet training. Anxieties about not performing these as practised earlier by that child, may lead to anxiety and possible incontinence as a result. One feature might be the emergence of obsessive behaviour. This may be manifested by increased preoccupation with toilet habits or cleanliness, such as hand-washing. All these or similar behaviours may be indications that there are problems and care is needed in the assessment of possible causes. Where such behaviours persist, the child may need to be seen by a psychologist who specialises in this area of child care.

## The 'phallic' stage (4–5 years)

From the age of about three to four years the next stage in Freud's consideration of psychosexual development is the 'phallic stage'. Associated with the phallus or penis, this period is the shift of preoccupation towards the genital area. All children are fascinated by differences in their anatomy and notice, early in life, differences between male and female. Freud described this period as being fraught with conflicting feelings towards parents, characterised by rivalry between themselves and parents of the opposite sex. There is also competitiveness for the attention of same sex parent. Freud used an analogy from Greek mythology, the story of Oedipus, to explain male sexuality and called it the **Oedipus complex**.

In the story Oedipus kills his father and unknowingly later marries his mother. According to Freud, a child unconsciously wishes to take his father's position as being the most important person in his mother's life. However, the child feels guilty at the awareness of these feelings and fears retaliation from his father. The unconscious defence mechanism that the child uses in order to reduce guilt and fear is called 'defensive identification'. This allows a stronger identification with the father and the masculine role, and a denial of feminine qualities and sexual feeling towards the mother. It also denies internal feelings associated with femininity, as at this stage of early, primitive defensive behaviour, the internal conflict has to be reduced by almost total assimilation of masculinity.

In girls the process is called the **Electra complex**. In this explanation of the development of female sexuality, the girl harbours feelings of attraction towards her father and competes with her mother for his attention. This may result in flirtatious behaviour towards her father as she attempts to usurp her mother for her father's affection. Again there is awareness and repression of these feelings, and eventually the girl identifies with the same sex parent.

There has been considerable criticism of Freud's theory of infantile sexuality. Karen Horney, for example, moved away from the orthodox Freudian view by disputing his psychological portrayal of women (Schultz and Schultz, 1994). Horney put more emphasis upon human relationships as significant factors in the development of personality, particularly that it is 'security' or a need for a secure relationship between people that motivates the individual, rather than just a sexual or aggressive drive.

More recently, there has been renewed interest arising from the accounts of child sexual abuse. Freud argued that the child's accusation of abuse, often levelled at the parents, was the result of 'fantasising' arising from the conflicting thoughts associated with this period of development. However, critics, particularly Masson (1989), have argued that Freud deliberately toned down the results of his clinical findings in order to protect his professional standing, particularly as many of his patients were the daughters of the rich and powerful in his community.

### Erikson's psychosocial stages

Unlike Freud, who stressed the biological determinism of behaviour, Erikson (1964) was interested in the effects of culture, such as parental influences, and societal influences in general. Erikson's view of human development is seen as the person progressing through eight stages of 'crisis', that is, developmental tasks that have to be completed before moving on – psychosocial stages (Fig. 3.2).

The first stage occurs from birth to 12–18 months, and is quintessentially concerned with the beginnings of *'trust'*. According to Erikson this early stage revolves around feeding. In Freud's view, feeding was described as a source of oral gratification, whereas Erikson took the view that feeding, while biologically essential, is the crucial theatre of interactions where the infant learns to trust and rely on his mother for security. Thus reliance, dependence and trustworthiness are gradually developed, and the child develops an 'inner certainty' that allows the growth of a sense of 'identity' and an ability to cope with moments of anxiety during which the child experiences being alone.

This theory helps to explain the possible reasons for differences in a child's ability to experience 'separation' from parents, and stressful

| Stage | Age | Characteristic |
|-------|-----|----------------|
| Trust versus mistrust | 0–15 months | Beginning of trust developing, learning to receive attention and feel wanted and loved. Failure results in difficulties in trusting in later life |
| Autonomy versus shame/doubt | 15 months–3 years | Sense of 'self' begins to develop, attempts to assert 'own will' on world, differentiation from parents. Failure results in poor self-confidence |
| Initiative versus guilt | 3–5 years | Development of sufficient self-confidence to 'explore' surrounding world, testing of limits. Failure results in withdrawal, guilt and obsessiveness. |

**Fig. 3.2**  Erikson's psychosocial life stages from birth to 5 years.

events such as hospitalisation. It is also an indicator of the ability to develop relationships with staff and other children.

From an interpersonal skills perspective, the child who has great difficulty adjusting to the separation from parents requires much more information about what is happening. This means comforting and holding the child much more often and assisting the child to trust that the health carer is 'telling the truth'. For this reason it is even more vital that whatever is promised is followed through. So, for example, a comment such as 'I will be with you in just a minute!' will begin to inculcate feelings of trust in such a child if the carer does attend in a minute! For a small child (and sometimes for adults) a minute can seem like a long time.

The next stage is called *'autonomy versus doubt'*, occurring between the ages of 18 months to 3 years. As the child grows and develops emotionally, the sense of 'self' and trust in others begins to grow. The awareness of 'self-will' and the ability to affect parents' behaviour increases, and the child will try to assert himself more and more. This is sometimes encapsulated by the phrase *'the terrible two's'* which describes the tantrums and truculent behaviour that can be seen in frustrated children of this age group.

Erikson's observations of childhood behaviour led him to note that despite increasing autonomy the child is still very dependent upon parents for love and security. Thus the child also has a sense of shame and doubt about behaviour that does not produce a warm response from parents. Erikson argued that a balance has to be achieved between limits which are acceptable and responsible and freedom to explore the world. Health carers will recognise the extreme frustration that children in this age range can express. However, the gradual progression from a passive infant to a restless and 'strong-willed toddler' is a normal one and indicates healthy development. Thus the two- or three-year-old who becomes withdrawn or unusually quiet and passive needs to be carefully observed, particularly where this behaviour is not readily associated with obvious physical cause.

The next 'crisis' in this approach is the period Erikson called '*Initiative versus guilt*'. This occurs from the age of three to five years and evolves gradually from the previous stage. It is essentially a deepening of the split between the part of the child's personality that desires to experiment and extend the boundaries of experience and the internal needs of the child for protection and approval. All children require approval and often go to extreme lengths to achieve this. Erikson argues for a harmony between permissiveness and the setting of limits. There is a distinction between allowing a child freedom to explore the world around them, and the freedom that has clear boundaries around what is safe and unsafe. In the clinical setting this may manifest itself by the child wanting to help the staff, often imitating behaviour, and seeking approval.

### Attachment theory

A number of significant ideas were developed during the 1900s related to the ways in which babies and children form attachments to their parents or care-givers and the effects of separation at various stages of development. Some of the key research was carried out notably by John Bowlby (1951), Konrad Lorenz (1966), Harlow and Harlow (1965), and Michael Rutter (1972).

Konrad Lorenz received a Nobel Prize for his ethological work on the behaviour of animals. Ethology is the study of animal behaviour through direct observation. Lorenz was very interested in the way in which young geese fix attention on the first thing that moves, immediately after their birth. For example the chick will follow around whatever it sees move, as soon as it is hatched. There is some original film of Lorenz being followed by a line of goslings who associated him as their 'mother'. Lorenz called this characteristic '*imprinting*', and argued that it was necessary for animals to react in such a spontaneous way for survival. Animals are capable of rapid physical development after birth, as compared with humans, who take many years of growth and nurture before maturity.

Harlow and Harlow (1965) set up experiments which demonstrated the importance of contact and comfort as part of attachment behaviour. Baby rhesus monkeys were raised with 'surrogate' or artificial mothers. These artificial mothers had the same shape as a real rhesus monkey, and were made of different materials. Some were formed from chicken wire and others with soft 'terry' towelling. The infant monkeys preferred the soft towelled surrogate and seemed to cling to this when frightened. The Harlows concluded that the monkeys had a psychological need for comfort, which they called *contact hunger*.

Human infants also have a need to be in close, warm contact with another person, which is why it is important to give hugs, to touch and give as much physical contact as possible during the child's time in hospital. Parents may become intimidated by the technology, or be frightened by it, and therefore may need encouragement to offer this. The interpersonal skill of holding and touching can therefore be practised as often as possible, either by direct involvement with the child, or by helping the parents hold the child as often as is practicable.

During infancy the child is considered to be reaching out for sensory experiences which assist in the differentiation between self and the outside world. Children who are denied sufficient stimulation or whose stimulation is restricted due to illness, can be severely affected by this, and may not develop the motivation for discovery and exploration. They become unable to interact or relate with the outside world if this condition is allowed to continue for long periods. There is much evidence from the studies gained from situations where children have been institutionalised, that deprivation of stimulation due to decreased adult–child interaction can lead to severe developmental problems (Rutter, 1972).

Bowlby (1951) was a psychotherapist working in London with parents and children who had emotional problems, due mainly to the effects of traumatic separation. These were essentially due to the Second World War, or the effects of long-term illness. According to Bowlby it is essential for the emotional development of the child, that the child should maintain a close and continuous relationship with the mother. He went as far as to argue that any psychiatric disorder always shows an incapacity for natural 'affectional bonding' and that such disorders in adult life have their roots in the disturbance of **attachment** during childhood (Bowlby, quoted in Rutter, 1972, p. 11).

He argued that:

> 'mother love in infancy and childhood is as important for mental health as are vitamins and proteins for physical health'.

> (Bowlby, 1951)

This view has of course influenced many practices in the care of children and the interpersonal behaviour of care-givers since his work was published. In a major review of the literature since the 1950s Rutter (1972) surveyed the work and critically examined the meaning of 'maternal deprivation'. He looked closely at what was meant by so-called 'quality mothering'. Rutter was able to make more distinctions between the various kinds of deprivation, distinguishing between a failure 'to make bonds' and deprivation after the bond has been made, thus suggesting that there are very different responses to separation depending on when and how the separation occurs.

He also went further than Bowlby by questioning the importance of the 'mother–child bond'. While arguing that this was of course highly important, he suggested that bonds made by the child with other adults during early development were also of significance. This may also account for the child's ability to cope with separation from mother and that children have an ability to form attachments with more than one person.

According to the attachment theory, a child that requires continuous care in hospital, develops, over a period of time, a syndrome called *hospitalism*. This is characterised by three progressive stages of:

- *protest*
- *despair*
- *denial.*

In a classic situation this would be manifested by anger and crying, calling for mother (protest). As the period of hospitalisation continues, the child becomes subdued and then becomes withdrawn. It is during this stage that he may develop the characteristics described above, of regressing in toilet habits, refusing food or attention (despair). He eventually, after repeated visits from his mother and family, becomes seemingly tolerant towards the situation. However, the next stage is the development of extreme detachment. On superficial observation the child appears happy and self-sufficient, but disinterested in any closeness (denial). He may become hostile towards his parents and engage better with the hospital staff. According to Bowlby, in this last stage the child has entered a phase where there is a serious breakdown in the primary attachment bond (Fraiberg, 1959).

When this occurs the parents need to be aware of this process and supported by staff. The most effective instruction is to inform the parents to remain consistently loving and supportive. Gradually he may then adjust and recover from the traumatic effects of the separation.

This explains the changes in attitude towards visiting that has occurred only since the 1960s. Parent accommodation is now being built in close proximity to the children's hospital, with parents now sleeping next to, or even with the child.

More recent research into the effects of separation has concluded that the child is not necessarily damaged by periods of prolonged separation when there is high quality care given by the parent substitutes (Siegelman and Shaffer, 1995, p. 422). 'Quality' in this context appears to be related to the amount of contact and interaction occurring between the adult and the child, where there is an atmosphere of warmth and responsiveness towards the children.

One of the principal differences between caring for adults and children is in the more active involvement of the parents in the care. Involving parents or family-centred care is not a new concept. Roy (1967) introduced 'active parenting' as a development of this idea using the principles of 'role theory' to assist parents in hospital settings (Saunders, 1994). In this approach the parents are actively involved in the care of their children, being taught and encouraged by staff. Such approaches are often very challenging to both carers and parents; judgements have to be made of how much the parents are able to tolerate in terms of involvement, in what may be distressing for them.

In the past, care has been focused on the individual, and family interventions have been largely ignored (Rennick, 1995). This has led to some staff resistance of open visiting and early parenting interventions (Saunders, 1994). The difficulty for staff may result in four types of interpersonal response, identified by Dixon (1993).

First, the carer may adopt a 'facilitative' approach recognising the parents' role in the care of the sick child. This results in giving support and removing barriers. Or second, the carer may become threatened by this 'encroachment' on the nature of the practitioner–child relationship, and the resultant behaviour becomes one of control over the parents and the enforcement of rules. The third alternative behaviour is where the health professional develops a relationship of trust and mutuality with the parents in which the parents are considered to be the experts in the care of their child. Fourth, avoidance behaviour, particularly where the parent becomes demanding or expresses different views to the staff concerning care, may develop.

It is possible to understand the above behaviours by relating them to the psychological defence mechanisms described by Freud (see Chapter 2). Having an anxious parent working alongside, in the care of a sick child, is stressful. The parent will require emotional support, explanation, teaching, reassurance and understanding. There is the added complication of dealing with this situation as well as caring for the sick child. It becomes possible to see why there is resistance to such a policy of care. Where the health professional is not given the support of senior colleagues in recognising such challenges, then coping by becoming more controlling toward the parent may result. Such controlling behaviour is often an unconscious way of dealing with internal feelings of not being able to deal effectively with the situation. It does bring some temporary relief, however usually leads to tension and the escalation of the stressful situation, with unhappiness to both carer and parent when conflict results.

Avoidance is a classic defence against the anxiety-provoking situation. It may be very deliberate at times, but is more likely to be an automatic and unhealthy defence against actively dealing with the pressure, and often leads to projection. This is where the carer 'dissociates' her own internal inadequacy and awareness of the difficulties, and projects inner feelings of anger and hostility on to the parent or other staff. Recognising that these internal feelings do not accord with her own notions of the 'ideal practitioner' who should be able to cope, the feelings are 'denied' and the situation is avoided.

In nursing practice, Saunders (1994) suggests a number of strategies that may help staff to adapt better interaction with parents in the care of children in intensive care units. These include:

- Accepting the centrality of the parents in making effective interventions with the nurse.
- Provision for feedback for the staff on how to make the relationship between nurse–parent and nurse–child, be the best possible, by discussing the challenges in an open way.

The interpersonal skills involved in utilising the above ideas can be considered as beginning with the development of the skill of looking for defensive behaviour in the both self, child and in the parents. The specific skills are then concerned with the attempt to interpret the behaviour in terms of the 'mental defence mechanism' that is being applied. For example, one can listen intently not only to what the parent is expressing about a sick child, but also to how it is being said. If there is anger, it may be important to acknowledge the cause, to accept the 'projection' rather than to collude or unwittingly ignore the emotion. Offering reassurance is a particularly important interpersonal skill, which can only be offered once the carer has actually identified the nature of the distress. Psychodynamic approaches do not assume the cause; the skill is to attempt to 'check out' the probable questions being asked with what is not being asked, and then to attempt to offer the most effective response. It is often obvious that a carer's answer to a question by an anxious parent does not seem to supply the 'desired response'. The skill of reassuring does not always mean giving the correct factual answer. Often it is acknowledging with the patient or parent, the unfairness of the situation, helping the other to see that you understand how they may be feeling.

## The person-centred approach

In Chapter 2 the centrality of the concept of the 'self' was described and the way in which the growing person develops a sense of personal identity. Such approaches have made significant contributions in promoting child-rearing practices. This approach, unlike the 'stage-orientated' determinism of the psychodynamic theorists, stresses the importance of the uniqueness of the child and the potential for positive growth. There are no specific developmental phases that the child enters; however, a broad distinction is made between the phase of growth before and after adolescence (Gething *et al.*, 1989). Much of the theory on which this approach is based assumes that the individual can know their phenomenological world. This means what is apparent to the senses and what is perceived and experienced by the person, rather than what the external reality actually is. There is an attempt to try to understand the child's actual experience rather than to think of the child like a mini-adult.

Such approaches are very similar philosophically to the educational development espoused by John Dewey (1916), the American educationalist who has influenced a more liberal approach to teaching young children. His methods encouraged the child to receive individual experiences which were developed through dialogue *with* the child rather than *to* the child. Such activities were to be guided by the teacher, not forced. Dewey has been very influential in changing attitudes about the child's ability to become self-directive and these have filtered into the practical approaches to caring. Practical examples of this process would include encouraging the child and family to undertake as much self-care as early as possible. Person-centred approaches involve the whole family in the process of care. This may include friends or even the family pet, where practicable, in the total care plan.

A consideration of specific interpersonal skills involved in the care of children suggests that there are specific types of communication needed in caring for children (Jolly, 1984). Jolly argues that while the act of communicating with children is often very imprecise, it is also the case that children have a higher level of understanding than they are given credit for.

In addition to the recommendation that carers must be honest and direct with children, several authors have taken this point further and suggested expanding the explanations given to children during hospital procedures to include 'telling the child where, when and how much pain they would experience', and describing other sensations the child may experience (Bates and Broome, 1986; Pridham *et al.*, 1987; Broome, 1990; quoted in Brennan, 1994).

Thus an important skill is in 'giving information' in such a way that it is accurate, avoids patronising, and gives sufficient detail that anxiety and some control over events can be taken by the child. An account of getting this wrong is described by Richard at the beginning of this chapter. He very honestly describes how an attempt to explain using simple language was misjudged. It is often a difficult skill to get right. Some children will be frightened of learning too much about a medical procedure, therefore the carer has to attend closely to the reaction and response in the child. However, in the majority of cases, giving information about what is going to happen has a positive effect in reducing anxiety.

In Chapter 2, Maslow's hierarchy of needs was described, and how such needs were organised by him as a way of understanding human motivation. In this explanation of human behaviour it can be seen that once the basic, fundamental physiological needs have been met, the child will require 'safety' needs to be satisfied. The following case example illustrates this.

*Clinical example*

Nina, a bright and lively eight-year-old, was admitted to the children's ward for an appendectomy early on Monday morning. Symptoms had developed gradually during the previous day, becoming more severe by Sunday evening. At first her parents had thought that she had a 'stomach bug' as she was complaining of 'griping pains and sickness'. Eventually the family GP was called and she was admitted for surgery, following a diagnosis of acute appendicitis.

On admission, Nina was pyrexial, in acute pain, nauseous and vomiting. It was clear that the family were very anxious. Nina was only able to communicate in grunts and groans at this point, and had been vomiting continuously since around 5 PM that day. Following examination by the surgical team she was admitted for surgery in the morning and prescribed sedation and analgesia and an intravenous infusion.

After half an hour Nina settled and, her physiological condition now stabilised, was able to get some rest as she felt very exhausted. Her parents, relieved that their daughter's condition was now being treated, felt less anxious, but were now concerned to understand more about the operative procedure booked for the next morning. The medical staff were able to explain what would happen and Nina's mother signed the consent form for the treatment to be performed. Nina's father took Nina's younger sister home and her mother stayed in the ward during the remainder of the night.

The next morning the surgery went ahead as scheduled at 8.30 AM and there were no complications. Nina's mother went to the anaesthetic room with her daughter and stayed with her until the she was induced. The staff were able to comfort Nina's mother and support her during this phase of treatment. Nina was returned to the ward by 10.30 AM, very drowsy and sleepy, but recognised her mother as soon as she came out of the anaesthetic.

The next day Nina was much more alert and sat out by her bed for lunch. Although feeling very tender, her appetite had returned and she was taking oral fluids well. The intravenous infusion of normal saline was removed, just before lunch and her temperature had returned to normal. Nina was now concerned about being away from home, and her 'pet cat, and sister'! Clearly there was anxiety now about how long she would be in hospital. There was relief when the nursing staff were able to explain both to her and to her family that she may be well enough to go home the next day, if her temperature remained normal overnight.

Nina felt much better, but later was able to express her fears to the nurse about having to have more 'injections' and wanted to know what would happen to her next, before going home. The staff were able to explain to both Nina and her parents that very few 'injections' were given now, analgesia being given through the intravenous line.

Later that night, as the night staff were settling her down, she was clearly wanting to help the staff as much as possible and to understand what they wanted her to do. It was clearly important to Nina that the staff liked her and felt that she was a 'good patient', so she tried very hard to comply with their requests. The next morning, her temperature remained 'normal', and the medical staff told her she could go home that day.

From this example it can be seen that at first the priority in Nina's care was to attend to the physiological needs. It was evident that she was in pain, dehydrated due to continuous vomiting, and very anxious; therefore treatment consisted of pain management, sedation to enable her some rest, and replacement of fluids by intravenous infusion. It was also possible to introduce analgesia and sedation via this route. This enabled the surgery to be carried out the next morning.

Once these needs had been met, and Nina was feeling better, she was then concerned about more fundamental 'security' needs. Feeling unsafe in this new environment into which she had been suddenly thrown as a result of her condition, she attempted to try to adapt to the milieu of the ward by introducing aspects of her home into the conversations. There was a wish to be 'at home', to feel safe around familiar objects like her 'pets'. Then as she became more aware of her situation and as the previous more 'basic' needs had been met, she began to want to 'fit in' to her new environment, to make friends with the nursing staff and be liked by them.

All of these very fundamental human needs were arranged by Maslow in his hierarchical order of importance which, depending on the circumstances, require satisfaction before the next level of need is perceived. Thus if a family is starving in a third world country, scraping grains of rice from the earth, they are not so concerned with being liked, and attending to their self-esteem.

In the clinical setting the nurse can use this model as a way of anticipating the needs of the child during the phases of care. Talking about home life, pets, brothers and sisters, can help the child to feel closer. Many staff wrongly feel that they had better avoid talking about home 'in case it makes the loss worse'. On the contrary, acknowledging the loss and talking openly about it with the child is often very helpful.

The health professional has a responsibility to work with the parents to allow the child to continue to develop, during hospitalisation or during a period of ill health. This may be very difficult when the child's care requires quiet and rest and they want to run around and play! In this case the nurse will need to set firm limits on behaviour and ensure a consistent approach is adopted. Some strategies will be discussed later when considering 'behavioural approaches'. At this age of course the child will not be content to walk, but will jump skip and climb wherever he or she can. An important consideration therefore for the nurse, is play.

The healthy child will be effervescent and full of ideas. During periods of ill health and debility the child will obviously be lacking the usual zestfulness but will still have an inquiring mind and, depending on the clinical circumstances, will become easily bored. As in Richard's account at the beginning of this chapter, staff may have to deal with a possible stream of questions. At the same time they have to deal with each child's health and appraise what he or she is capable of doing. Allowing time to play is part of the child's developmental needs. It may only be possible for a child to play while lying in bed. One of the challenges of nursing children is the ability to keep up with the child's ideas. Statements made by children often require a response. For example the child may make a number of observations such as 'today I saw a bus ... there's the doctor ... I played on the slide'. These statements require an answer and are an important part of child development (Fraiberg, 1959).

Play is vital to effective communication and crucial for healthy mental development. It is the way in which children make sense of the world and rehearse interventions with others. It has been described as the 'laboratory in which the child learns to master their environment' (Craft and Denehy, 1990, p. 94; Fig. 3.3). Play is used by care staff as a therapeutic intervention. It therefore requires planning, devising specific objectives beforehand, followed by careful evaluation.

The well-equipped area for play activity should contain not only the usual collection of toys and drawing equipment but also 'dressing up' materials which enable the children to role-play their experience in hospital. Examples of such items include old bandages, toy syringes, stethoscopes, nurses and doctors gowns, uniforms, and any other items the carer can think of that encourage children to simulate their current situation. It may become evident by playing with a child how they are affected by their own hospitalisation. Care must be taken by staff not to 'overinterpret' the situation; however, observing and talking to the child during such role-play activity can provide important information and facilitate intervention.

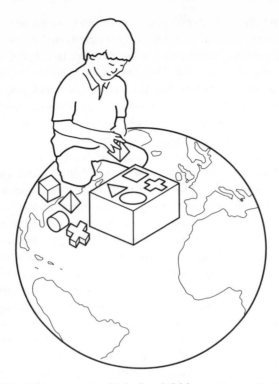

**Fig. 3.3**  Play: 'the laboratory in which the child learns to master their environment' (Craft and Denehy, 1990)

Researchers have also cautioned against too much emphasis on 'organised', planned play activity (Bolig, 1990; Doverty, 1992). They argue that therapeutic play can not replace unstructured play for the child, and that health carers must never attempt to be too directive and must ensure a balance between the two activities.

Because all but the most physically unwell child will have the energy to want to undertake some activity, and because of the high degree of stress that hospitalisation creates, most children will rapidly engage in therapeutic play. Nevertheless, staff have to provide the occasion for the child to play, and be able to plan their own time to join in the activity. The child will be able to detect 'pressurised time', when the carer is trying to give attention but has her mind elsewhere! Thus the importance of planning. (This is not to deny that at times the involvement can be spontaneous; however, such involvement usually does occur in some 'window of opportunity' during which the carer is relaxed.)

The child is likely to be anxious and perhaps regress as a result of feeling vulnerable, therefore the choice of toys or objects may be 'below' the expected age level. This is a natural response to the stressful situation and does not necessarily mean more serious psychological problems. Evaluation consists of reporting back to the health care team the observations and any other relevant information that may be important in the general consideration of that child's overall care.

# Behavioural approaches

For the health professional the significance of a child's dependence upon the adult for security is of importance. It is for this reason that clear instructions about what is permissible and what is not, is fundamentally important. The child in hospital is very vulnerable, taken away from the routines of home life and placed in a completely alien environment.

The behavioural approach focuses attention on learning and interventions are much more structured. Positive and negative reinforcements (see Chapter 2) are used to increase desired behaviour and decrease undesired patterns of behaviour, respectively. It remains primarily the parents' responsibility for matters of discipline and control; however, the health team may need to advise them, especially during such stressful periods as the hospitalisation of their child. This begins with the carer giving attention to the words she is using during explanations or instructions. For example the use of the words 'good' or 'bad', may be used unwittingly: it may connote behaviour that the child is intended to perform. However, for the child such words can be perceived as having other implications (Stanford, 1991). As children may believe that their illness is punishment for 'bad' behaviour, use of such words may increase this belief (Brennan, 1994).

Clearly there has to be a balance between allowing a child freedom, and the need to promote immobility and rest for therapeutic reasons. This is the area of care that can be the most trying for the health team. Behavioural approaches can be very helpful in this respect. The therapeutic approach requires careful and consistent planning and must be applied by the whole team if it is to be successful. This may be particularly the case in community settings. Hospitalised children are usually more subdued as they are more acutely ill.

## *Limit-setting*

The interpersonal skill of ***limit-setting*** can be very useful in this context. It is based upon the behavioural process of 'reinforcement'. Any person who has had to undergo a hospital procedure will know that it is important to understand what is expected and to be briefed on what to expect. For the child this becomes even more significant and can often reduce the level of anxiety, particularly where some control is allowed. For example, the older child may feel more secure if allowed to squeeze the carer's hand, with the instructions to squeeze when ready to begin, and to squeeze again when a 'break' is needed. There is some evidence that this provides security, when the child is feeling vulnerable and fearful; being told what to do and how to behave can reduce other fantasies about being out of control (Gohsman, 1981). The child is thus 'held' emotionally by the prescribed behaviour directed by the carer. Care must be taken not to offer too much choice during times of stress as this can often increase the tension.

*Clinical example*

In terms of the child's behaviour, the 'acceptable' must be stated again in a firm and clear way and must be enforced. An example might be where a particular environment has a 'rule' that all children must rest between 2 PM and 3.30 PM, and that this is a 'ground rule'. To be successful this has to be enforced by all staff, and the carer has to ensure that there are clear instructions and an agreed policy.

Next it has to be communicated clearly to all children so that the expectation is explicit. Where a child tries to 'break' this rule there must be clear understanding of the sanctions which can be used. For example there may be 'grounding' the child from some treat to be shared by the other children – ice creams, sweets, or other treats that can be used as 'reinforcers'. When the child does accept the rule and conforms in the desired way then such treats can be used to positively reinforce the desired behaviour. Such methods have to be discussed with the parents, and can be used collaboratively with the family.

Setting limits also means that the carer expresses clearly and firmly the behaviour that is acceptable. An effective way of dealing with the child who perhaps wants to undertake some activity which is contrary to advised instruction, is to attempt to negotiate a compromise. For example it might be telling a child that they 'cannot get out of bed now but they will be allowed out for extra time if they stay there for 60 minutes' (or whatever)! It is important that this is followed through if the child eventually acquiesces. Other positive treats and rewards can be given out to increase desired behaviour and this is frequently performed by carers working with children. Some clinical areas use 'bravery awards' and 'star charts' which offer a system of reward for behaviour. Such conventions can, however, be controversial: a child may, for example, suppress expressing pain if he is wanting to get attention in this way.

## Caring for the dying child

The carer will at intervals have to care for the dying child. This is a very distressing area for many staff and requires special interpersonal skills in helping the patient and the family.

Children become very aware of death at quite an early age. Clearly, how each child comprehends the detail of this fact varies according to age and maturity. It is believed that children up to the age of two years have little or no comprehension; however, this may differ according to how the child has been socialised and also the child's cultural background. It is therefore important for the carer to assess the child and family individually, rather than assume a specific age-related fixed point at which an awareness and understanding of death emerges.

Caring for the dying child is an aspect of child care which is often difficult to accept. It is never accepted within society, particularly western societies. Health care staff may feel the powerlessness of the situation profoundly. Learning how to effectively care for the dying child means understanding the grief process, which itself requires an awareness of the relationship between grief and attachment. As described earlier in this chapter, Bowlby's theory of attachment describes the human propensity to make strong affectional ties. When these ties are broken there is a strong emotional reaction. The stages that any person goes through are similar, only varying in intensity depending on the cause of the loss, feelings being obviously more intense when the loss is for another human being. The common experiences of loss are:

- *feelings of anxiety*
- *anger*
- *depression*
- *detachment.*

Bowlby (1981) suggested that there were more similarities than differences between adult and childhood grieving, and later added a phase called 'numbing' that both he and Parkes (1972) had observed in children. Thus the stages were refined to include the following.

- *Numbing* which is characterised by feelings of disbelief, disorientation and shock. Often there may be accompanying feelings of panic or anxiety.
- *Yearning and searching* for the lost person. This may go on for an indefinite period; sometimes it has been known to go on for years.
- *Insomnia and restlessness*, with cycles of sobbing and distress, which seem to overcome the person in waves of intensity.
- *Anger* is a common feature. This may be directed towards the staff, towards parents or projected on to the lost person for 'causing the grief' or abandonment.

The child may feel guilt at these ambivalent feelings and may feel the cause of all the distress. Interpersonal skills applied in such situations begin with the carer listening to the child (or the parents), and not interrupting. Facile reassurance is not helpful and usually only serves to make the carer feel better. What is usually more effective is to listen carefully to the feelings being expressed; allow them to be fully ventilated rather than be 'cut off'. It is then important to present reality gently, that the child 'is not being punished for some past misdeed' or that the 'parents are not to blame, that they have done all they can, and that it is not their fault that this has happened to their child'. It may be appropriate to put them in touch with organisations where they may receive support from others with similar experiences; however, this should not be rushed or offered too soon.

One of the common fears staff experience is that of impotence and powerlessness, characterised by an inability to think of appropriate responses to make, therefore the carer may avoid the situation. This may be further compounded by the carer's own 'guilt' about having failed the child and his parents. These feelings are experienced by most health care staff at some time in their careers.

Once the numbing disorientation of the immediate grief begins to pass, there is often a time of conflict and turmoil, of 'aching grief', labile emotions and wretched self-recrimination. The best intervention the carer can make is a calm presence, sitting with the family, or the child, and demonstrating with them a willingness to understand the grief and provide support and comfort through presence and time. From an interpersonal perspective this means taking cues from the situation and talking when the child or family wants to express feelings, and remaining silent but present (that is, alert to the reality of the situation, the non-verbal signals) and responding as honestly as possible to what is asked. Dealing honestly with questions from both child and parents may be the source of uncomfortable feelings of dissonance for the caring staff.

Sound 'person-centred' approaches suggest that the best therapeutic method is honesty and genuineness. However at times this creates an ethical dilemma; for example the child may not know that he has a terminal condition and asks questions about when he will get better, or the parents may still be awaiting the outcome of investigations for their child, who the health care team suspect to be suffering from a terminal condition. Such situations become the real tests of how to retain dignity and integrity in everyday practice and maintain appropriate professionalism as part of a team, sharing the difficulties. Some children intuitively seem to know that they are dying, but seem to pretend that they are well in order to protect their parents. When health carers notice this may be happening they can assist the child, who may be very frightened, by becoming the key adult who they can talk to about their fears.

The answers to these dilemmas are only to be found in the constant discussion with the team and with the clinical supervisor or mentor. There are never 'black and white', clearly written protocols which guide all practice. The overriding consideration has to be the welfare of the patient and the family, in a trusting and honest way, when dealing with the limitations of treatment and care. This at times means breaking bad news and being realistic about the limits of personal abilities. That is to accept that the carer is also human. Crying with the family in times of grief is not an indication of unsound practice. It is often another way of sharing the grief with the family.

If, however, the carer finds herself to be very distraught over the death of a child and feels her grief is overpowering and preventing the family from engaging in their own loss, then she needs to be aware of what is happening and withdraw temporarily from the scene. It is important that care is handed over to another who can, at that moment, attend to the family. This is an example of a professional and considered intervention, which indicates maturity and awareness.

## Summary

Interpersonal skills are essentially part of the overall repertoire of skills required to care for sick children. It is particularly pertinent in this area. Communicating clearly and effectively is not just a matter of learning to listen and respond. While these form part of good practice, it is also vital that the carer is aware of the theoretical underpinnings to the interventions she is using. This increases confidence in knowing when and how to respond, and enables informed alternatives to be used when tried interventions fail.

Health carers provide 24-hour care for the child and his family and therefore have the most contact with them. This significantly contributes to a better understanding of how the child and family are progressing and reacting to the clinical interventions.

Understanding the psychodynamic reactions as defences against pain and fear, embarrassment and poor self-esteem, provide ways of interpreting the behaviour in such a way that helping strategies can be planned, based upon sound understanding of the processes involved.

Awareness of the 'person-centred' approaches to care assists in developing a trusting relationship of non-possessive control with the family. Behavioural techniques based upon reinforcement of desired behaviour, when used judicially, can be effective in helping to deal with challenging behaviour in the child.

Research has demonstrated that both psychological and physiological variables can create pain, discomfort, anxiety and affect care outcomes. The role of health professionals in this area of care is to be alert to the value system of the family (Hinson, 1985, p. 63), and be open to understanding the context from which the child comes. This includes an attempt to understand and respond to the family's conflicts and behaviour patterns.

# References

Bates, T.A. and Broome, M. (1986) Preparation of children for hospitalisation and surgery: a review of the literature. *Journal of Paediatric Nursing* 1, 230–39.

Benner, P. and Tanner, C. (1987) Clinical judgement: how expert nurses use intuition. *American Journal of Nursing* 87 (1), 23–31.

Bolig, R. (1990) Play in health care settings: a challenge for the 1990s. *Children's Health Care* 19, 229–33.

Bowlby, J. (1951) *Maternal Care and Mental Health*. World Health Organisation, Geneva.

Bowlby, J. (1981) *Loss*. Penguin Books, Middlesex.

Brennan, A. (1994) Caring for children during procedures: a review of the literature. *Pediatric Nursing* 20 No. 5, September/October 1994, 451–58.

Broome, M.E. (1986) The relationship between children's fears and behaviour during a painful event. *Children's Health Care* 14, 142–45.

Broome, M.E. (1990) Preparation of children for painful procedures. *Pediatric Nursing* 16, 537–41.

Craft, M.J. and Denehy, J.A. (1990) *Nursing Interventions for Infants and Children.* WB Saunders Co., Philadelphia, USA.

D'Apolito, K. (1991) What is an organised infant? *Neonatal Network* **10**(1), 23–33.

Dewey, J. (1916) *Democracy in Education.* MacMillan, New York.

Dixon, D.M. (1993) Parent participation during hospitalisation: Understanding differences. In Saunders, A.N. (1994) Changing nurse's attitudes toward parenting in NICU. *Pediatric Nursing* **20**, No. 4, July/August, 392–94.

Doverty, N. (1992) Therapeutic use of play in hospitals. *British Journal of Nursing* **1**, 77–81.

Erikson, E.H. (1964) *Childhood and Society.* Norton, New York.

Fraiberg, S.H. (1959) *The Magic Years.* Methuen, London.

Freud, S. (1905) *Three Essays on Sexuality,* standard edn, Vol. XII. Hogarth, London.

Gething, L., Hachard, D., Papalia, D.E. and Olds, S.W. (1989) *Life Span Development.* McGraw-Hill Book Company, Sydney.

Gohsman, B. (1981) The hospitalised child and the need for mastery. *Issues in Comprehensive Paediatric Care* **5**, 65–76.

Goldson, E. (1992) The neonatal intensive care unit: premature infants and parents. *Infants and young children* **4**(3), 31–42.

Harlow, H.F. and Harlow, M. (1965) The affectional systems. In *Behaviour of Non-Human Primates,* Vol. 11, (eds A. Schrier, H. Harlow and W. Stollnitz). Academic Press, New York.

Hinson, F. (1985) *Handbook of Paediatric Nursing.* Williams & Williams, Adis Pty Ltd, Sydney.

Jolly, J. (1984) *The Other Side of Paediatrics.* MacMillan Press Ltd, London.

Lorenz, K.Z. (1966) *On Aggression.* Harcourt Brace Jovanovich, New York.

Masson, J. (1989) *Against Therapy.* Fontana/Collins, London.

Parkes, C.M. (1972) *Bereavement.* Penguin Books, Middlesex.

Perrin, E.C. and Gerrity, P.S. (1981) There's a demon in your belly: children's understanding of illness. *Pediatrics* **69**, 841–49.

Piaget, J. (1977) *The Development of Thought: Equilibrium of Cognitive Structures.* The Viking Press, New York.

Pridham, K.F., Adelson, F. and Hansen, M.F. (1987) Helping children deal with procedures in a clinic setting: a developmental approach. *Journal of Paediatric Nursing* **2**, 13–22.

Rayner, E. (1993) *Human Development: An Introduction to the Psychodynamics of Growth, Maturity and Ageing,* 3rd edn. Routledge, London.

Rennick, J.E. (1995) The changing profile of acute childhood illness: a need for the development of family nursing knowledge. *Journal of Advanced Nursing* **22**, 258–66.

Roy, S.M.C. (1967) Role cues and mothers of hospitalised children. *Nursing Research* **16**, 178–82.

Rutter, M. (1972) *Maternal Deprivation Reassessed.* Penguin Books, Middlesex.

Saunders, A.N. (1994) Changing nurses' attitudes toward parenting in NICU. *Pediatric Nursing* **20**, No. 4, July/August, 392–94.

Schultz, D. and Schultz, S.E. (1994) *Theories of Personality.* Brookes-Cole Publications, California, USA.

Siegelman, C.K. and Shaffer, D.R. (1995) *Life-Span Development*, 2nd edn. Brookes-Cole Publications, California, USA.

Stanford, G. (1991) Beyond honesty: choosing language for talking to children about pain and procedures. *Children's Health Care* **20**, 261–62.

Stanley, J.M. and Moore, R.S. (1995) Therapeutic effects of music and mother's voice on premature infants. *Pediatric Nursing* **21**, No. 6, November/December.

Wolff, P.H. (1969) The natural history of crying and other vocalizations in early infancy. In *Determinants of Infant Behaviour* Vol. 4 (B.M. Foss, ed.). Methuen, London.

# Further reading

Carter, B. and Dearmun, A.K. (1995) *Child Health Care Nursing: Concepts, Theory, and Practice*. Blackwell Science, Oxford.

Freud, S. (1915) *Introductory Lectures on Psychoanalysis*, standard edn, Vol. XV. Hogarth and Harmondsworth: Penguin, London.

Freud, S. (1923) *The Ego and the Id*, standard edn, Vol. XXIII. Hogarth and Harmondsworth: Penguin, London.

Klaus, M.H. and Kennell, J.H. (1982) *Parent–Infant Bonding*. Mosby, Chicago, USA.

Roberts, M. and Tamburri, J. (1981) *Child Development 0–5*. Holmes McDougal, London.

# Chapter 4
# Approaches to Care in Adolescence

This chapter begins with an account by a student occupational therapist who describes her work with adolescent patients. It is a frank and open recollection of both the highs and lows of her experiences with this age group. The chapter then develops theoretical ideas, exploring the three approaches used in this book and relating them to the issues affecting the adolescent in care. An attempt has been made to explore key areas that affect the adolescent, such as eating disorders and dealing with the angry patient.

*Maria, a student occupational therapist*

'As a student occupational therapist, I have worked in several clinical settings, with a variety of client age groups. One of the most challenging is working with the adolescent client. Adolescence is a very imprecise term: opinion seems to be divided as to what age a child enters the mysteries of this period of development. However, for me there are clearly observable differences to be seen in children around the age of 11–12 years. The child becomes more self-conscious and more aware of the opposite sex! I have found working with this age group very demanding on my ability to be creative.

I recall working with a young teenager called Rachel who was suffering from a chronic condition and I was taking part in an assessment. We were attempting to establish a joint plan of activities to help the client from becoming bored and frustrated during a lengthy phase of treatment following treatment for burns. It proved to be an extremely tense series of meetings, with the client turning down every possible suggestion for assistance and spending time alone in her room. While this was an understandable reaction to her condition, her records suggested that she had always adapted very well and had a 'lively and extrovert personality'.

It was clear that we needed to investigate whether Rachel was becoming depressed, as she became detached and morose. I attempted to ask how she was feeling and at first this did not seem to have any significant effect. However, as I persisted I felt she was beginning to trust me more, and a rapport developed. Gradually Rachel talked about her condition and her feelings about this. Although fed up, she appeared to be accepting what had happened, but complained of being bored with hospital routine. I tried to find out what her interests were.

Given her age I felt sure she would be interested in popular music. As I was only recently out of my teens myself, I felt sure this would work. Unfortunately she expressed no enthusiasm to my enquiries about the music charts, various bands or the music scene in general. Books, films, current affairs, cookery – nothing seemed to be of interest to her. Until one day I mentioned the staff nurse on the ward who was renovating an old sports car. At this piece of news her 'ears seemed to prick up' and she suddenly became animated, asking me questions about the car . . . "what sort of car, how old . . . what make and model?".

I had stumbled on this client's passionate interest and I brought in some car magazines for her. Her parents, whom we had asked to help us, did not know anything about this new interest, which had only recently developed.

Having now established a focus of interest we were then able to develop the relationship. The interest in old cars worked well and we were able to set up projects, areas of study and skill development together. We were able to persuade the staff nurse to take her to visit his car and for her to see for herself some of the restoration.

After this discovery Rachel seemed like a totally different person.

Clearly there are a number of factors involved in this story other than just adolescence. Chronic clinical conditions create mood swings and it is possible in such circumstances to develop depression. However, in this instance there were no obvious signs of clinical depression, that is the client was eating and sleeping quite normally, her parents just felt that she had become very 'sensitive' and more prone to periods of withdrawal, anger and general tetchiness. This description, together with the pattern of behaviour we were seeing, seemed to be more like adolescent withdrawal rather than the development of a depressive response.

While adults respond in angry or irritable ways in similar circumstances, usually it is not so prolonged. Angry or tetchy outbursts seem to be more spontaneous or impulsive, unless the client is becoming withdrawn and depressed. I have also found that adults can be encouraged to talk about their feelings or be helped to do so. With more life experience adults can usually find more appropriate words to describe their reactions. Adolescents are less confident about expressing themselves.

I can clearly remember my periods of withdrawal and irritability as a teenager, believing that adults were 'ancient' and really knew little about my feelings, or about what was important to me. Keeping this in mind when dealing with this age group is helpful to me in preserving tolerance and understanding.

Defining the precise age of adolescence is not helpful, as Maria suggests in the above account. It is more important to acknowledge a 'transitional period' that exists between childhood and adulthood. Adolescence is a period of gradual and intensive physical and psychosocial development. Physically it embraces the period of puberty, which for girls may begin at the age of eight or nine years, and in boys perhaps a few years later. Adolescence is commonly thought to end at around the age of 18 years (Bee, 1994). However, individual changes such as personality, stability, or maturity vary immensely. Socially there are many differences too, with some individuals married with children by the time they are 18 years old. Therefore cultural variations also affect notions of what this period actually consists of. For Adrian Mole it was waking up one morning covered in red spots (Townsend, 1982).

Hamberg (1974) summed up this period as having three major events.

- Biological changes, occurring as a result of hormonal changes and creating sudden development. The adolescent seems to 'shoot up' overnight and acquires adult height.
- Psychological and social changes. The adolescent associates much more with his peers, has a growing interest in self-image and accompanying concerns about self-identity.
- Role changes which these two factors produce. These changes are mainly related to peer and family relationships.

J.D. Salinger's (1958) *The Catcher in the Rye* provides an excellent description of the above changes. The opening paragraph begins with an adolescent's view of his childhood and relationship with his family.

## Health and adolescence

There are a specific number of health issues that are related to this age group. Adolescence, despite all the mental and physical changes that occur, is actually a time of less acute illness than at other periods in the life span. However, traumatic events, death and accident rates rise during this stage of life. Most of these are due to motor vehicle accidents, and increasingly where this occurs the victim has been intoxicated with alcohol.

Anorexia nervosa and bulimia are conditions which are significantly higher in this group and seem to be increasing (Bee, 1994). Both conditions are associated with eating behaviour and are characterised by excessive concern with weight and weight loss. Health workers are very likely to encounter this condition, or know of a family affected by this disorder. Current estimates do vary, but most researchers agree that at least 5%, with as many as 18% of teenage girls, are bulimic (Millstein and Litt, 1990).

Suicide is another serious risk in this age group. Rates have increased since 1960 and now represent around 15% of deaths in teenage years (Hawton, 1986). There are also disturbing differences in suicide rates in differing parts of the world; for example, Australia has a very high youth suicide rate, as well as death from major trauma (WHO, 1986).

In a Canadian study, Bibby and Posterski (1992) surveyed 4000 adolescents and discovered that 63% believed adults did not understand them, and 71% believed adults did not have confidence in them. Rosenbaum and Carty (1996) argue that it is important for health professionals to have some understanding of the 'meanings and experiences of adolescence, within their subculture'. This means attempting to understand the language and issues of importance to the adolescent in order to be in the best position to give 'culturally relevant care'. One study (Rosenbaum and Carty, 1996) asks three fundamental questions.

1. What is the meaning of 'care' to adolescents within family and their peer subculture?
2. What does 'health' mean to them?
3. How does 'care' contribute to the health of adolescents?

The researchers found several themes emerging from the study. First, for the adolescent, care meant *'being there'*, this meaning that the adult can be relied upon to listen with sincerity, 'giving them a hug and saying they are important to you'. Second, 'clothes, hair and music' are important as 'metaphors' for the adolescent's emerging identity. According to the study, clothes emphasise the inter-generational differences. Wearing jeans and not looking like adults help to encourage a separate identity. Music was considered to be a way of making a similar statement. Disapproving parental tastes in music was seen as being part of a distinction between adolescent and adult.

For girls the onset of adolescence occurs around puberty, with appearance of breasts, widening of the hips and menstruation. These changes have historically been treated with fear and superstition. If the family situation allows open discussion of bodily functioning and children are encouraged to ask questions about their sex and bodily functioning, the transition for the adolescent is usually natural and without great anxiety. However, many families still treat this transition in development as a taboo area. Menstruation was regarded in the past as 'the curse'. With it the girl often had anxieties about internal functioning, bleeding and 'mess'. Of course it also symbolises the fact that 'babies can now be produced'. Raynor (1993), describes how this can lead to an explosion of sexual feelings which may be perceived as pleasant, disgusting or frightening, depending on the way the girl has been brought up.

For boys this period is also a time of high sexual excitement and arousal. Girls are usually the cause of ambivalent feelings and to cope with the confusion boys normally group together and jeer at the girls as a way of dealing with their feelings (Raynor, 1993).

Working with adolescents is therefore affected by personal attitudes to development and sexuality, requiring the helper to be aware of their own embarrassment and to openly confront fears and questions that may arise. For example, adolescence is a time of intense auto-erotic self-stimulation. Raynor (1993) argues that from a psychodynamic perspective, masturbation is a release of adolescent rage and release of frustration. It also helps discovery of one's own body and 'brings its image closer to images of other bodies'. Thus it is a natural part of sexual development which eventually leads to the development of a relationship. Respecting the adolescent's privacy, knocking on doors before entering the room and generally acknowledging this phase in the client's development may lead to the prevention of embarrassment.

Adolescence is also a time when 'idealisations' occur. This is the passionate hero worship which leads to interest in pop and film stars and can become very intense. Sometimes it can be transferred on to members of staff. Usually this is harmless and transitory; however, when it does develop into infatuation the staff member has to take care to respect the client's feelings and treat the situation seriously. This may require talking through the relationship and gently affirming the 'professional' boundary, while at the same time reassuring the client that they are still 'very good friends'. Some helpers have great difficulty in confronting such situations and often choose to ignore the client as an alternative way of dealing with the situation. This is not a very therapeutic way of handling it and may be seen by the client as quite uncaring and hurtful. It has to be stressed that for the adolescent who requires hospital care, or is ill, the internal turmoil natural to this part of life becomes even more frightening and out of control. Thus intense attraction to others who display concern and caring is often powerful.

## Psychodynamic perspectives

Erikson's (1958) view of this stage of development focuses very much upon the development of a sense of *identity*. He characterises this stage as 'identity versus role confusion' (Fig. 4.1). He argues that the adolescent is constantly attempting to appraise changing ideas and experiences, and adapt the emerging sense of self. Erikson views this stage as occurring between the ages of 13 to 18 years of age. His ideas have been very influential within psychology and education for expanding the understanding of adolescence. Erikson argues that in order to arrive at a mature self-identity, the adolescent must re-examine the roles he must occupy. For example, in a social setting the adolescent may find himself at a gathering where he is no longer perceived as a child and cannot therefore play with the younger children, but neither is he an adult, lacking the experience to join in the 'adult conversation'. Most of us can recall such awkward moments. The confusion that Erikson refers to is the result of exposure to a rapidly changing set of expectations from others and an attempt to blend into the 'main group'. For the adolescent this is not always a very easy accomplishment. Add to this the typical

| Approximate age | Nature of change | Activity of the stage |
|---|---|---|
| 13–18 years | Identity versus role confusion | Quest for acceptance and search for new values. Transition from childhood to acceptance as an adult |

Fig. 4.1   Erikson's psychosocial stages in adolescence.

drop in self-esteem which accompanies this stage and at times adolescent life can be very uncomfortable (Harter, 1990). Maria describes these feelings quite well in the account of her own behaviour, where she describes thinking of adults as being 'ancient and unable to understand her'.

It is with the peer group that the adolescent finds expression and support. For this reason hospitalisation or prolonged periods of ill health can be very disruptive. Marcia (1980) has developed Erikson's work on identity formation. He suggests two components: *crisis* and *commitment*. It is for this reason, Erikson suggests, that adolescents develop fixed views about others, being particularly intolerant towards those who are perceived to be different. It becomes a defence against the sense of identity confusion that the adolescent experiences at this stage of life (Erikson, 1980).

A crisis in this context means a period of decision-making, when old values or ways of thinking have to be challenged by the individual and reassessed. The outcome of this process is a commitment to behave in a different way. This may be an abrupt or gradual change. Any 'challenge' to health at this time is a clear crisis that requires considerable adaptation. This is true for any person; however, it is more acute in the adolescent period. There may be a sudden switch into childlike regression as a result of overwhelming fears or stoical indifference to what is happening. In attempting to work therapeutically the carer may observe both these extremes of behaviour and be flexible enough to recognise what is happening. Clear explanations and well-thought-through education of the patient are fundamentally important in this area of health care practice.

Loevinger (1976) builds upon the psychodynamic view of ego development (see Chapter 2), viewing each stage as a 'radical restructuring' of the adolescent's relationship to life and to the world. Loevinger argues that the adolescent reaches a *'conformist' stage*, where he sees himself in terms of his membership of a group, such as family, school, religious or music group. In the group his sense of belonging and identity is defined, and a strong intolerance to anything perceived as being outside of the group is assumed.

Gradually the adolescent becomes more self-aware and, rather than perceiving authority as being inflicted from the external world, a 'them or us' association, it becomes transformed into a more mature, sensitive view of the world where 'authority' becomes 'internalised'. Here the individual creates his own internal standards and attempts to live by this code of conduct. Although shaped by his upbringing, parents, school and society, he now perceives himself as part of a world he shares with others. Loevinger describes this as the *conscientious stage*.

An example of the 'conformist' stage, is the young adolescent who feels that his parents are constantly 'at him'! He feels persecuted by them when they ask him 'to clear up after him, to think of others and not just himself'. However, a gradual change in his behaviour occurs and he begins to notice the outside world, for instance choosing to go against possible family values connected with food and embrace vegetarianism. It is at this stage that he may begin to develop a passionate interest in the welfare of others and the planet around him.

## Eating disorders

There are a number of potential theories about the cause of eating disorder, and these are mainly inconclusive. Some of these range from theories of abnormal brain functioning (Leibowitz, 1983) to purely psychosociological ideas about the construction of identity by the media and society at large (Orbach, 1988).

From a psychodynamic view disorders such as anorexia and bulimia have complex aetiologies (Bee, 1994) which are associated with the powerful image of food. Clinical anorexia nervosa presents as a morbid preoccupation with the calorific value of food and an obsessive denial of any food intake which if ingested would cause fattening. The desire of the sufferer is to be ultra-thin, with the individual perceiving self as fatter than he or she is in reality. Associated with the condition are feelings of failure and depression.

The *control* which accompanies the denial of food may be a significant element. This has led researchers to suggest that anorexics have a fear of growing up, of achieving adult identity and responsibility; the psycho-dynamic mechanisms of *repression, displacement* and *conversion* therefore forming the basic mechanisms in this disorder. All of the fear associated with 'growing up' becomes 'repressed' in the mind of the adolescent, who then, through the process of 'displacing' the anxieties, becomes obsessed with control through the withholding of food and a preoccupation with the physical state ('conversion' of the psychological fear into a more manageable physical manifestation).

These 'fears' related to growing are very complex and are not, as is commonly mistaken, clichéd ideas about the adolescent wishing to stay in a Peter Pan world of childhood. Often there are considerable issues related to the child feeling unable to control what is happening. The above mechanisms, which are unconsciously applied, may become a way out in the adolescent's mind.

Anorexia is predominantly a condition affecting young women aged between 12 to 18 years. If the patient continues to starve themselves, menstruation (which may have only recently commenced) stops. This is argued by some writers as further evidence that the individual is attempting to halt growing into adulthood. The psychodynamic mechanism is *regression,* or reverting to earlier more childlike patterns of behaviour as a reaction to extreme stress. It must be pointed out that these ideas are purely speculative.

In the author's experience of working with patients with this disorder, the features are varied in how they are expressed by different individuals from differing family backgrounds. The condition is likely to have a number of possible predisposing factors. However the psychodynamic explanations do allow consideration of the individual dynamics in more depth.

Food itself is steeped in metaphor and symbolism. Ambrosia was the food of the gods in classical mythology. A cake is baked as a token of affection or as a symbol of celebration. It has always been a tradition to bring a sick person gifts of fruit or other consumable delicacies when visiting in hospital. Refusing food can sometimes be associated with a rebuttal or a signal of contempt. On visits to friends or relatives it is usual to be offered tea, biscuits or cake. To refuse an enthusiastic offer is often difficult.

Anorexia is a symbolic self-denial which verges on self-abuse. This is particularly so with the condition *bulimia nervosa,* which consists of more frequent episodes of binge eating and systematic self-induced purging. In practice a fine line may exist between the two conditions described here, with patients often exhibiting symptoms of both conditions at times. A key feature is secretiveness, so the disorder may have been present for some time without the family being aware. The onset of major weight loss, or in some cases attempts at suicide, indicates the presence of a serious condition. Depression and the risk of suicide attempts are always present because of the severe self-loathing which is always a feature of the disorder. It is possible to regard this condition as an insidious suicide attempt, a kind of self-inflicted 'failure to thrive', a prolonged self-cannibalism. Eating disorders are very disruptive conditions, with much self-directed anger, either towards the self or towards the adult world.

Using the psychodynamic approach is like attempting to be a detective, considering possible motives and testing how this may relate to the individual circumstances. It is for this reason that this approach is often criticised as being purely 'interpretive' and non-scientific. Exploring the 'secondary gain' patients may derive from their behaviour is helpful for the health professional. It provides a way of questioning which may help throw light on to the way a patient is really feeling.

The interpersonal skills required to care for patients with this condition are built upon an understanding of the above unconscious processes. Caring for the adolescent with eating disorder is often very disturbing and trying, and requires persistence and the development of a clear understanding between carer and patient. Treatment regimes vary; however, as the focus of treatment in the early stages will be to address the physical components of the disorder, the carer can play an important role in allowing the patient to express anger and fear.

The degree of distress that is experienced will of course be related to the severity of the condition. With some patients the carer can be helpful by exploring the patient's 'self-identity', that is, the emerging view of 'self' in relation to others. Careful observation of interpersonal relationships with family, staff and other patients can help the carer to build up a better appreciation of the possible dynamics involved. Using the therapeutic relationship to assist the development of self-confidence in the patient is an important area in this context. This can be facilitated through encouragement to talk about personal fears, giving appropriate praise and exploring how feelings of control can be re-evaluated.

While these areas take time and may necessarily take place over a longer period of time, the carer using psychodynamic understanding can help to identify which mechanisms may be involved in the condition.

The development of a trusting relationship between carer and adolescent may take time. Although the need for a relationship in which there is support and awareness of need is present, the adolescent may appear to be suspicious. It is for this reason that working therapeutically means setting up firm limits about what is acceptable behaviour and what is expected of the client. If the helper waivers and changes expectations too much, the client will feel uncared for. From a psycho-dynamic view this behaviour has its origins in childhood uncertainty, and the anxiety created by feeling alone. From a behavioural viewpoint, the helper tackles the anxiety in a more direct way.

## Behavioural approaches

The adolescent will often engage in 'testing the limits', finding out through continuous challenging of authority 'how far he can go'. This behaviour requires a united approach from the whole health care team, as any variation among staff will create the potential for confusion and manipulation of staff. This is important, because the carer, in an attempt to communicate concern may be tempted to 'give in' to the adolescent who is testing the limits, without realising what is actually going on. When this contributes to the adolescent feeling he can easily manipulate the helpers it will raise his doubts and delay, rather than build, a good rapport.

Setting firm limits implies a strict, disciplinary approach. This is not the case. What is intended is the creation of *security* through a consistent approach, by making a concerted effort to establish agreed team decision-making, in regard to the patient's behaviour. For Maria, in the opening account, this meant offering rewards such as a visit to see the restoration work on the car. This was agreed as a part of the 'contract' only as a result of more cooperation with her treatment.

Consider the following case story.

*Clinical example – Susan*

Susan is a bright 13-year-old who had insulin-dependent diabetes which had developed six months previously. Diabetes is one of the most common endocrine disorders of childhood and adolescence (Kyngas *et al.*, 1996). It is a chronic condition, associated with insulin insufficiency and requiring a lifelong regime of daily insulin injections, attention to regular diet and exercise.

Susan was admitted to the children's hospital for regulation of her regime which had become erratic. Her recent history indicated rows with parents over the management of her insulin and diet. On several occasions she had become confused and disorientated and had been taken to the local casualty department for treatment. Staff found this to be due to either not eating her prescribed diet for that time of day, for example missing breakfast or lunch, or delaying the time of her insulin injections.

On admission she appeared quiet and morose most of the time. Her insulin and diet were reviewed and found to need some minor alterations to dose and intake respectively. Education and advice were offered by the team which included dieticians and staff she knew from the insulin clinic she regularly attended.

However Carol, an occupational therapist working with Susan in the ward, began to notice she would ask each member of staff the same question. For example, on one occasion Susan asked a staff nurse, a junior doctor and a nursing assistant what time lunch was, as she was 'popping to the hospital shop to buy some stamps'. Consequently she arrived back late for her meal. When Carol again began to explain the implications of missing regular meals Susan immediately explained that she had asked about meal times but had received 'three different times' from staff. Thus she was able to successfully 'play one member of staff off against the other'. This behaviour continued and at every opportunity she tested the limits and concerns of the staff in whatever way she could, even withholding her self-administered injections until a member of staff reminded or asked her to do so.

It was decided to ensure that the staff each had a very clear strategy for responding, which meant setting up a contract for medication and meals at preset times, and getting her to agree to these times. This was translated into a written chart which Susan was responsible for signing. Rewards, in the way of praise or other treats, were offered, for example choosing CDs or videos from the library. This worked very well and soon Susan's behaviour changed; she began to behave in a more responsible way to her treatment regime.

Later Carol was able to talk to her about what was going on. At first Susan denied that there had ever been a problem, however gradually felt able to talk about a number of issues that had bothered her. These included her fears about having the condition, and she also 'blamed her parents', for having diabetes. Also, she felt frightened and lacked confidence in feeling that she could manage her condition on her own. This fear conflicted fiercely with a need to 'do things on her own and not be constantly nagged by adults'. Carol was able to reassure Susan that these feelings were quite natural and that feeling anger was perfectly understandable. Susan benefited from making friends with other teenagers who were also coming to terms with diabetes.

This case example highlights the importance of involving the patient in the treatment regime as much as possible and ensuring that care is jointly planned, with complete understanding and mutual agreement reached. Behavioural approaches are linked to '*rewards*', which is why many health workers find it a mechanistic way of dealing with others. However, behavioural methods often underlie the approach used to deal with difficult situations encountered in practice.

Rewards are important considerations in behavioural approaches. Desired behaviour, that is behaviour that is not harmful to the patient or to others, is rewarded. Antisocial or undesirable behaviour is ignored;

the theoretical assumption being that when the individual seeks attention and reward, this behaviour can then be encouraged.

Behavioural-based care has to be carefully planned. Careful assessment of the problem occurs as an integral part of the process. This means
collecting details of the behaviour that is unacceptable and, importantly,
how the client perceives it. In this context 'behaviour' has a wide variety
of meanings. For instance it may refer to anxious responses of a patient
to their treatment, or being simply naughty, for example refusing to
attend schooling, or refusing other parts of the care plan. If appeals to
reason and careful explanation fail, behavioural techniques can be
assessed as a viable way of changing behaviour. This begins with
finding a suitable 'reward'. Threats to exclude or withdraw the client
from the 'rewarding' situations must be carried out so that the patient
knows staff mean what they say! Thereafter, any slight change for the
better is immediately rewarded, so careful vigilance by staff for signs of
improvement must be observed.

The emphasis is on careful *assessment* of the behaviour with the
patient. Planning can then proceed 'with' the patient and, where possible with his agreement. At times cooperation will not be possible.
Through careful assessment it is still possible to find some reward which
will have meaning for the patient, which can be used to encourage the
desired behaviour. Collection of all available information will allow staff
to produce a specifically tailored plan which will always consist of a
reward that is likely to motivate change. Failure to do so is usually
linked to the reward being insufficient to produce the required change.

Hostility and verbal aggression can be dealt with by using behavioural approaches. Behavioural approaches have concentrated upon
the ways in which the aggressive individual has learnt inappropriate
ways of dealing with frustration or aggressive feelings. In the 1930s a
team of behaviourists concluded that all aggression is created by frustration (Sdorow, 1995, p. 643). The theory developed was called the
*frustration–aggression hypothesis*. This suggested that anger results
from the blocking of a goal. Berkowitz (1974) later revised this theory,
suggesting that while this does not always result in an aggressive out-
burst, it may produce other unpleasant emotions, such as anxiety or
depression. Where a patient may behave in a constantly aggressive way,
a careful behavioural programme can be very effective. The plan will
have to include a clear description of the behaviour, gently confronting
the patient with what is unacceptable and jointly planning more
acceptable ways of communicating with staff.

Lack of attention from health care staff is often a main contributor of angry exchanges in the adolescent. Setting clear limits of times during the day when staff will attend to the patient or relatives, and being explicit about carrying this through, is often an effective and simple way of diffusing anger.

The following account will deal more specifically with a person's verbal anger and discuss methods or techniques for handling the situation. While a number of methods and techniques have been developed to deal with physical aggression, little work has been carried out on dealing with verbal abuse. Self and Viau (1980), suggest *four steps* for helping patients alleviate anger:

1. identification of the anger
2. acceptance/acknowledgement of the patient's anger
3. exploration of the anger
4. channelling the anger.

This method, however, assumes that the patient *wishes to understand their anger*. It does not help the carer with the majority of situations she faces, where patients do not wish to be analytical at that time!

Another attempt was made by Sandford (1985) who describes techniques such as allowing the protagonist the right to their view and questioning in an attempt to understand the real cause of the anger.

While there are no 'magical' solutions, the author has developed *five basic techniques* which have been validated for health workers and shown to have a positive effect in helping to deal with such outbursts (Wondrak and Dolan, 1992; Fig. 4.2). The techniques are:

1. side-stepping
2. self-disclosure
3. partial agreement
4. gentle confrontation
5. being specific.

## Side-stepping

In this technique the aim is to respond in a totally non-defensive way to the provocation (which is often very difficult to do). It is also an appropriate device to use when exposed to an unexpected verbal attack. The technique is to indicate that you have heard what the patient has said without becoming hooked into it, basically assuming that the adolescent is angry and that you can understand the reason for the

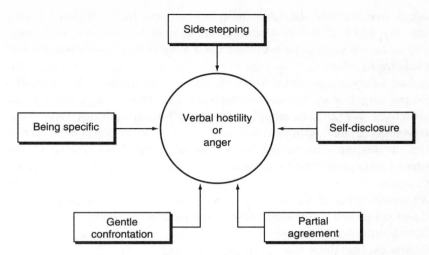

**Fig. 4.2**   Five techniques for dealing with verbal anger or hostility (Wondrak and Dolan, 1992).

frustration, however at the same time avoiding becoming enmeshed in argument and becoming defensive. For example:

Protagonist: 'Call yourself a carer – you are useless. I've been waiting all morning for someone to see to me, and all I been told is "We will be with you shortly!!"'
Carer: 'Yes you are correct, it has been busy. But I am free now to help you'.

This example was chosen as it is a common scenario. Many health staff become defensive and try to explain and then defend how busy the staff have been. This may not be the best way of dealing with the anger. Giving the reasons may be appropriate later; however, at that time a more direct approach is called for. This technique seeks to prevent the situation from getting out of control. The carer needs to offer some compromise. If it is not possible to help at that moment, it may be possible to give an accurate indication of when you can deal with the situation. Giving information and attention helps to reduce frustration.

### Self-disclosure

Used sensibly this technique can help the carer by reducing the anxiety of entering a discussion with someone who is angry or verbally aggressive. Health staff can often be trapped into responding in a stereotypical way, offering jargonised answers. Instead of a more open and honest response they project what they may think is required of them in an attempt to be seen as 'in control' or efficient. Rather than respond in this way it may be more appropriate for the carer to tell the protagonist that she is upset by his anger, perhaps using a statement such as 'I feel nervous when . . .' or 'I feel I cannot get through to you when you shout/are so angry'.

This technique has to be limited to what the carer is able to feel comfortable with. When the carer is truly upset by what a patient threatens, unable to think of what to say, it may give some time for self-composure. It is also an appropriate response with adolescents because they may be able to identify with the response more readily, or else may not be sufficiently aware of how upsetting their comments may be. Giving this feedback may at times be helpful.

## Partial agreement

This is a powerful technique which is useful for dealing with hostile criticism from others. By agreeing with part of the criticism, however not *all* of it, the possibility opens for maintenance of the carer's self-esteem.

### Clinical example

Carol, a junior student nurse, is working in a children's clinical area where she is to care for John. John has a serious condition which requires long-term treatment. He becomes very irritable during the prolonged periods of care and has a tendency to let his anger out on the staff. He can also be very cutting and has upset a number of junior carers who he feels are too incompetent to be able to care for him. On this occasion he confronts Carol: 'You don't know anything about my condition do you . . . how can they let people train as nurses when they don't even know basic things about dialysis'.

Carol replies: 'Well I am a student nurse and am therefore learning – no one can claim to be an expert in all areas, John! Although I can see it may be difficult for you to have to continually meet new staff'.

The aim of 'partial agreement' is to respond positively and not treat the remarks as an accusation, even if that is how they are intended. This technique seeks to be a way of reducing hostility. At times, however, a more direct confrontation may be the only option!

This may be the case where the carer experiences sexual harassment. Many health workers feel that it is inappropriate to deal with an incident at work in the same way they would a similar incident outside of work. This attitude needs to be challenged. Working in a health care setting does not give licence to patients to abuse the carer, or for the carer to act like blotting paper, soaking up verbal abuse or harassment. Firm limits need to be set, as do clear statements about what is acceptable behaviour and what is not, so that this can then be upheld by the whole team. This is the only way such behaviour can be dealt with effectively.

## Gentle confrontation

This follows on from partial agreement as a technique. It aims to move the criticism from the personal to the more general and perhaps get at what may actually lie behind the anger. It can help to expose manipulation and constructively attempts to redirect the anger.

Consider the following interaction between a patient and a junior student nurse:

Patient: 'Just look at yourself ... how can you be expected to take care of me when you look like that? How do they allow staff to wear studs and rings in their faces and still be professional?'

Carer: 'I can see that you disapprove of the way I look. I'm not trying to offend you though and I would like to help you this morning.'

Patient: 'Well you are offending me ... fancy looking like that and expecting to be a nurse!'

Carer: 'I see your point. How I look does not affect my skills though ... you seem to be very angry and upset and that must be awful. Are you worried about anything else?'

As can be seen from this example the carer acknowledges how the patient may be feeing but does not attempt to be drawn in to a discussion of the superficial content. Instead she wonders if the patient's anger may be related to something else, or perhaps to feelings of safety and apprehension about being cared for.

## Being specific

This is a technique which is quite difficult to perform in stressful situations. With practice it can be helpful. Decide what you want to say and say it as simply as possible. The skill is to avoid unnecessary padding and come to the point quickly. This way it is much more likely to be heard by the patient who may only be able to take in small details due to their excited emotional state.

These techniques have been developed as a way of equipping the health worker with simple 'tools' which may, in the event of being confronted by a hostile or aggressive verbal attack, promote a more therapeutic and de-escalating process. Thus by attempting to raise consciousness and avoid the carer becoming defensive and retaliating, the situation is defused (Wondrak, 1989).

# Person-centred approaches

The person-centred approach focuses on empowering the patient with as much control of treatment as possible. The three basic interpersonal elements of this approach are empathic intervention, genuineness and positive regard (see Chapter 2).

## *Empathy and identification*

Empathy is considered to be an essential feature of the effective patient–carer relationship (Baillie, 1996). It is defined as 'the ability to enter into the life of another person, to perceive his current feelings and their meanings' (Kalisch, 1973). This means attempting to understand how a situation affects the other person. The process involved is *'identification'*, an ability to relax 'self-control' of one's own perceptions, to attempt to see the other's situation. This is much easier to describe than actually practice, and unfortunately many health professionals need to be 'in control' in order to carry out their daily work.

Empathy is a skill that develops as the other person becomes better known and does not occur instantly! Sundeen *et al.* (1994, p. 176) argue that it is impossible to say 'I'm going to empathise with Mr Jones today!'. Empathic communication evolves as the relationship develops. Getting to 'know' the adolescent may take longer, because of the swings of mood which occur in this age group. Empathic understanding is a necessary component of trust. Travelbee has defined trust in this context as the:

'assured belief that the other individual is capable of assisting in times of distress, and will probably do so'.

(Travelbee, 1971)

The fundamental basis of trust is the high probability that others will assist in a 'crisis'. For the adolescent who is still testing out the reliability of other people, this may take longer.

## Genuineness

The health professional will find times when being 'genuine' with patients is very difficult. Many staff have experienced such difficulty due to failure to think through the consequences of their actions or words. In reality there are real restraints – the knowledge base, clinical policies and protocols which may inhibit the giving of information. More importantly, there are ethical issues concerning the information that a person may be able to cope with at once. This is not to *encourage* economy with the truth; however, a distinction has to be made between total openness and clinical responsibility. The basis of the relationship has to be upon the reality that there is a real inequality in the relationship between carer and patient, an unequal power relationship. Giving all available information will not necessarily empower the patient. If a patient asks for information it becomes the staff's responsibility to inform and educate as effectively as possible. However, some patients do not wish to know all the details. Being carefree about the information in such cases may be neglectful of the patient's actual needs and creates unnecessary anxiety.

In a social relationship a mutual sharing and openness exists which is quite different from the patient–carer relationship. This distinction needs to be considered by the carer. The basis of the person-centred approach is to improve the patient's ability to cope with their situation. At times it may be necessary to 'take charge', to be prescriptive and tell the patient what to do, which can create a feeling of safety for the patient. The skill is to develop an awareness of when the patient is able to take more personal responsibility.

## Positive regard

This notion is a worthy one: to treat everyone with the same tolerance and understanding, as individuals, irrespective of who they are or what they may have done (Rogers, 1975).

Support from health care staff is very important when working with adolescents (Thorne, 1990; Burroughs *et al.*, 1993). Adolescents are very astute and may feel that health care staff are guided by routine, rather than genuine interest in them as individuals (Hentinen and Kyngas,

1992). Nursing research has highlighted that when collecting information, for example during admission of an adolescent client, the focus is often on the patient's disease process (Brydolf and Segesten, 1996). The authors suggest asking about 'living conditions', such as describing a normal week, and then compare this to how the adolescent feels the condition affects them in the present circumstances. They argue that this can produce a wealth of new information of how the illness affects the patient in a personal way.

Positive regard is also associated with the term 'respect' which appears frequently in the health care literature. Respect can be defined as the giving of particular or 'special' attention. Browne (1993) reviews the use of the term and argues that respect is a 'primary nursing ethic' that must form the basis of all interpersonal relationships within the health domain.

In summary the three basic elements – empathic intervention, genuineness and positive regard – form the basis of most relationships. Rogers was raising the importance of the carer's responsibility to be self-aware and think carefully about the nature of the relationship with patients as a means of encouraging a more therapeutic outcome. The following case example illustrates this.

*Clinical example – Steven*

Steven was a bright 14-year-old who had been admitted for investigation of an abdominal swelling. He was alert and interested in what was happening to him but also seemed apprehensive about asking carers, particularly young female staff, about his condition. His parents visited daily and were very worried about him and the possible cause of the swelling. A number of tests were carried out during the first week of admission and several differential diagnoses were considered by the medical team. However there remained uncertainty about the precise cause.

Steven became aware of the uncertainty about the cause, not so much by what was said, but by the avoidance to tell him that there was an uncertainty. Staff were evasive. The battery of tests, which to the staff were mainly routine, consisted of X-rays, including barium swallows (where Steven swallowed flavoured drinks opaque to X-rays in an effort to diagnose internal abnormality), blood tests, and vigorous physical examinations by a number of medical experts.

Steven was informed about the need for tests but there was an avoidance of any detailed explanation about what was going on. While staff were concerned about keeping him informed and attempting to explain what was happening, the explanations were usually kept brief and generally fell to the most junior student nurse to answer. He later told a nurse that he felt awkward about staff seeing him naked or being with him when he undressed, which some staff had mistaken for anxiety associated with the actual investigative procedure. On one occasion, after several hours of barium swallow examination, he soiled his pyjamas on the way back to the ward but felt too embarrassed to tell anyone so he washed them out in the bathroom and returned to his bed with them damp.

While the staff were caring and intellectually aware of his potential embarrassment, they dealt with it instead by colluding. In other words, they pretended not to notice his embarrassment.

In the above account it is clear that more careful education and aware-ness may have helped both Steven and the staff. For example the staff could have outlined that soiling may occur as a consequence of a barium swallow, giving a more sensitively prepared introduction to the procedure. Spare pyjamas could have been left with him, and reassur-ance about both the method of barium swallow and possible effects may have helped to avoid his embarrassment. Developing empathy occurs over time. In this example it is clear that the carer can learn to deal with the situation differently.

Thinking about how the patient may be feeling, attempting to connect more with the *experience of the situation*, rather than the illness itself, helps to develop empathic understanding. Anderson (1981) found that 'emotional distancing', an attempt on behalf of the carer to cut off feelings, produces barriers to empathic understanding. The patient may feel uncared for or excluded. Such interpersonal communication is often conveyed in the carer's non-verbal behaviour, tone of voice, eye contact, use of touch, or use of silence.

Junior health care staff may be concentrating on getting the procedure performed accurately and may be neglecting the psychological state of the patient, for example neglecting eye contact and other indicators of the patient's mental status. Both are clearly necessary in order to show competence, technical ability and interpersonal awareness.

## Conclusions

Caring for the adolescent is a demanding and challenging area of health care. An ability to identify with the patient, imagining what the experience of illness means, is crucial to successful care. This means not only understanding the effects of the illness symptoms, but also the way in which the patient's everyday interaction and behaviour are affected.

The application of the 'psychodynamic' approach is helpful as a method of understanding the underlying anxiety the adolescent may experience in relation to his or her disorder. 'Client-centred' and 'behavioural' skills can be applied to deal with the anxiety and behaviour of the child.

The adolescent is at a very impressionable time of life. The carer must be prepared to work effectively as a 'role model', demonstrating skills in attending and listening. Be prepared to negotiate in the care planning process with the patient. Show tolerance and understanding, particularly in response to frustration and anger.

In order to carry out this formidable list of skills it is important that members of the health care team support each other. Clear lines of communication are necessary; all the team members need to ensure awareness of both individual and unit care policy. It is the responsibility of all staff to ensure they keep themselves aware and raise possible ambiguities at the appropriate staff meetings. Clinical managers can assist this process by encouraging regular support and clinical supervision, opportunities for staff to discuss clinical difficulties and review care plans.

# References

Anderson, N. (1981) Exclusion: a study of depersonalization in health care. *Journal of Humanistic Psychology* **21**, 67.

Baillie, L. (1996) A phenomenological study of the nature of empathy. *Journal of Advanced Nursing* **24**, 1300–308.

Bee, H. (1994) *Lifespan Development*. Harper Collins, New York.

Berkowitz, L. (1974) Some determinants of impulsive regression. *Psychological Review* **81**, 165–76.

Bibby, R.W. and Posterski, D.C. (1992) Teen Trends: A Nation in Motion. Stoddart, Toronto. In: Rosenbaum J.N. and Carty, L. (1996) The subculture of adolescence: beliefs and individuation within Leininger's theory. *Journal of Advanced Nursing* **23**, 731–46.

Browne, A. (1993) A conceptual clarification of respect. *Journal of Advanced Nursing* **18**(2), 211–17.

Brydolf, M. and Segesten, K. (1996) Living with ulcerative colitis: experiences of adolescents and young adults. *Journal of Advanced Nursing* **23**, 39–47.

Burroughs, T.E., Pontious, S.L. and Santiago, J.V. (1993) The relationship among six psychosocial domains, age, health care adherents, and metabolic control in adolescents with IDDM. *The Diabetic Educator* **19**, 396–402.

Erikson, E.H. (1980) *Identity and the Life Cycle*. Norton, New York.

Hamberg, B. (1974) Early adolescence: a specific and stressful stage of the life cycle. In *Coping and Adaptation* (eds G.V. Coelho, D.A. Hamberg and E. Adams). Basic Books, New York.

Harter, S. (1990) Processes underlying adolescent self concept formation. In *From Childhood to Adolescence: A Transitional Period?* (G.R. Adams and T.P. Gullotta, eds). Sage, Newbury Park, California.

Hawton, K. (1986) *Suicide and Attempted Suicide among Children and Adolescents*. Sage, Beverly Hills, California.

Hentinen, M. and Kyngas, H. (1992) Compliance of young diabetics with health care regimens. *Journal of Advanced Nursing* **17**, 530–36.

Kalisch, B. (1973) What is empathy? *American Journal of Nursing* **73**, 1548.

Kyngas, H., Hentinen, M., Koivukangas, P. and Ohinmaa, A. (1996) Young diabetics' compliance in the framework of the mimic model. *Journal of Advanced Nursing* **24**, 997–1005.

Leibowitz, S.F. (1983) Noradrenergic functions in the medial hypothalamus: potential relation to anorexia nervosa and bulimia. In *The Psychobiology of Anorexia Nervosa* (K.M. Perke and D. Ploog, eds). Springer, New York.

Loevinger, J. (1976) *Ego Development*. Jossey-Bass, San Francisco.

Marcia, J.E. (1980) Identity in adolescence. In *Handbook of Adolescent Psychology* (J. Adelson, ed.). Wiley, New York, 159–87.

Millstein, S.G. and Litt, I.R. (1990) Adolescent health. In *At the Threshold: The Developing Adolescent* (S.S. Feldman and G.R. Elliot, eds). Harvard University Press, Cambridge, Massachusetts.

Orbach, S. (1988) *Fat is a Feminist Issue*. Arrow, London.

Raynor, E. (1993) *Human Development*. Routledge, London.

Rogers, C. (1975) Empathic: an unappreciated way of being. *Counselling Psychologist* **5**(22), 2–10.

Rosenbaum, J.N. and Carty, L. (1996) The subculture of adolescence: beliefs and individuation within Leininger's theory. *Journal of Advanced Nursing* **23**, 731–46.

Salinger, J.D. *The Catcher in the Rye*. Penguin Books, London.

Sandford, K. (1985) How to cope with verbal abuse. *Nursing Life* **5**(5), Sept/ October. 52–55.

Sdorow, L.M. (1995) *Psychology*. WCB Brown & Benchmark Wm C Brown Communications Inc, Iowa.

Self, P.R. and Viau, J.J. (1980) Four steps for helping the patient alleviate anger. *Nursing (US)* **10**(12), 66.

Sundeen, S.J., Stuart, G.W., Rankin, E.A.D. and Cohen, S.A. (1994) *Nurse–Client Interaction*, 5th edn. Mosby, St Louis, Missouri.

Thorne, S.E. (1990) Constructive non-compliance in chronic illness. *Holistic Nursing Practice* **5**, 62–69.

Townsend, S. (1982), *The Secret Diary of Adrian Mole Aged Thirteen and Three Quarters*. Methuen, London.

Travelbee, C.B. (1971) *Interpersonal Aspects of Nursing*. F.A. Davis, Philadelphia.

Wondrak, R. (1989) Dealing with verbal abuse. *Nurse Education Today* **9**, 276–80.

Wondrak, R. and Dolan, B. (1992) Dealing with verbal abuse: an evaluation of the efficacy of a workshop for student nurses. *Nurse Education Today* **9**, 108–15.

World Health Organisation (1986) *Young peoples's health: a challenge for society.* Technical Report 731, WHO, Geneva.

# Further reading

Carter, B. and Dearmun, A.K. (1995) *Child Health Care Nursing: Concepts, Theory and Practice.* Blackwell Science, Oxford.

Feldman, S.S. and Elliot, G.R. (1990) (eds) *At the Threshold: The Developing Adolescent.* Harvard University Press, Cambridge, Massachusetts.

Taylor, J. and Muller, D. (1994) *Nursing Adolescents: Research and Psychological Perspectives.* Blackwell Science, Oxford.

# Chapter 5

# Approaches to the Care of the Adult

Throughout this book emphasis is put on the importance of listening carefully to what the patient is actually saying. 'Active listening' is a fundamental interpersonal skill. The narrative which follows, presents an adult patient's view of interactions with members of the caring team during a period of hospitalisation. It provides a view of how a patient makes sense of what is happening around him.

### A patient's account

'I had been admitted to the medical ward of my local hospital for investigations into the cause of a prolonged high temperature. The nurse described it as a "pyrexia of unknown origin". Earlier in the year I had travelled to eastern Asia, and a possible connection between this and my raging temperature had been raised by my general practitioner. I was admitted into a side room of the ward. After a week with a very high temperature and feeling ill, I was relieved to be going into hospital to find out what was wrong with me.

Over the next few days a number of investigations were carried out to find the cause. I had to produce a sputum sample and was given vigorous physiotherapy to loosen up the secretions. My raised temperature continued over several days while the medical staff investigated the cause. On one occasion the nurse jokingly commented, "Congratulations, you have the highest temperature on the ward", which I was not particularly proud of at that time! An intravenous infusion of fluid was prescribed by the medical staff as I was becoming dehydrated. Eventually the cause was discovered to be a "mico-virus" pneumonia, and I was prescribed the appropriate intravenous antibiotic.

During the four days of investigations I found that there were three main ways in which the staff approached me. While this is obviously a crude differentiation, the "types" described behaved very differently towards me.

The first approach I called the "techno-type". This represented the staff who seemed to interact with me via the apparatus I was attached to. So the intravenous tubing would be like an extension of me, and the staff would say hello and communicate with me via the tubing, checking and altering the rate and flow. Little eye contact took place, attention being directed at the technical apparatus.

The next approach I called "care-plan" orientated. Usually nurses, but other staff too, such as physiotherapists, would interact with me via the notes and charts that they either brought with them or pored over at the end of the bed. Communication was carried out mainly in regard to what seemed like "set" questions, for example checking my bowel habits, how many cups of tea I had to drink that morning. Again eye contact was minimal between me and the carer.

Finally, a carer approached me who was able to relate more directly to me as a person, as well as take care of the records and equipment around me. I called this carer the "intuitive type". For example, one day I was feeling very fatigued and unwell. My temperature was raised and I felt terrible. The carer had just come on duty and introduced herself as the "nurse caring for me that afternoon". She looked at me and noticed how ill and frightened I looked and told me she was going to help me to feel better. She helped me into the bathroom and ran a bowl of tepid water and helped me to sponge myself down, which felt very cooling. On returning to the bed she sat me in a chair next to the bed and noticed that the mattress was covered in a plastic cover. The nurse removed the plastic cover, replacing it with a cotton "draw-sheet" and fresh top sheet. Then she helped me back into bed and put fresh covers on the pillows. I did feel better; she helped to make me feel safe and cared for. I felt that she knew and understood how I was actually feeling, and communicated with me as a person feeling unwell, rather than as a "condition". This was very reassuring'.

Although the classification in the above discussion is simplistic, it does illustrate how carers can be perceived by patients and draws attention to the way in which it is possible to become professionally blinkered by the technology or theoretical approach. The patient's view of the care he received indicates how it is possible for the carer to become so absorbed by the task that the patient feels excluded.

# Health and adulthood

The period of adult life between the ages of 20 to 30 years has been described as 'demographically dense' (Rindfuss, 1991) because in this span there is more action in most people's lives than in any other period of the lifespan – more marriages, divorces, moves of house, births, employment and unemployment. Despite some 'spreading out' of these events due to increasing longevity, early adulthood is still the most active phase of life for most people. With this comes increased stress and associated health risks. However this period is also considered to be the time of optimum physical functioning, a time during which the body is at its physical peak.

Mortality in the young adult is more likely to be due to suicide, accident or homicide, than disease. Disease begins to contribute to causes of death in the late 30s and 40s, when heart disease and cancer begin to emerge as contributory causes (Bee, 1994). There is, however, growing evidence that health patterns in the adult show that the risk of emotional disorder is increasing in this age group, being highest in the 24- to 44-year-old period. The disorders include depression, anxiety disorders, substance abuse, and mental health disorders such as schizophrenia (Kessler *et al.*, 1992).

This chapter will focus on some of the main implications of working in a psychodynamic, behavioural or person-centred way with the adult patient. Care that has been known traditionally as 'general/adult' represents a very broad spectrum of activity. It can encompass cardiology, nephrology, neurology, medical and surgical areas. For clarity, this chapter refers to the 'adult' as a person between the ages of 18–65 years, receiving care in a variety of settings.

# Psychodynamic approaches

Erikson's (1980) stages of psychosocial development place emphasis on the importance of maintaining intimate relationships in the period of young adulthood. He describes the stage between the ages of 19–25 years as *intimacy versus despair*. Erikson defines this as the ability to establish a clear sense of who we are as individual beings, so that there is no fear of becoming emotionally involved in an intimate relationship with a partner. For example, during adolescence there is a need to separate from parental influence and increasingly learn to develop and trust one's own choices. For Erikson, intimacy with another in an adult relationship cannot occur until the individual has developed a clear sense of identity (Bee, 1994, p. 30; see also Chapter 2).

### Transference and counter-transference

Progression through Erikson's life stages occurs as a result of new social challenges in the person's life. The two key concepts of *transference* and *counter-transference* assist in understanding how people react to new social conditions.

Transference refers to the way in which the feelings, thoughts and actions of the patient are often unconsciously affected by his earlier childhood experiences. Counter-transference, as the name suggests, is the same phenomenon, in this instance affecting the carer, so that earlier experiences unconsciously affect the carer's perception of the patient (Fig. 5.1).

Holmes and Lindley (1991) suggest that transference can arise in two contexts.

- Everyday or 'fleeting' transference, whereby hopes and expectations impinge on the patient's interactions with the carer. An example would be the powerful way in which the doctor, nurse or therapist is perceived by the patient.
- 'Deep' transference whereby the patient may become besotted or unduly attracted to the carer.

All transference reactions are linked to associations with the past. This is usually towards parental figures who have had a significant effect upon the person's formative development. Most individuals can recall a significant person, possibly at school, or certainly in early adolescent life, who had a significant impact upon them. This may have been either a positive or negative effect. Later in life, during stressful situations, these positive or negative feelings may suddenly become unconsciously attached to people in the immediate situation. It is important to stress the totally unconscious nature in which this occurs. There is no conscious awareness of these feelings, thoughts or actions being 'transferred', the mechanism being 'automatic'. Hospitalisation is an example of where vulnerability, produced by ill health, can often trigger powerful transference reactions. The carer can do more than just be aware of this process or note when it occurs. It is possible to work with the transference in a positive way.

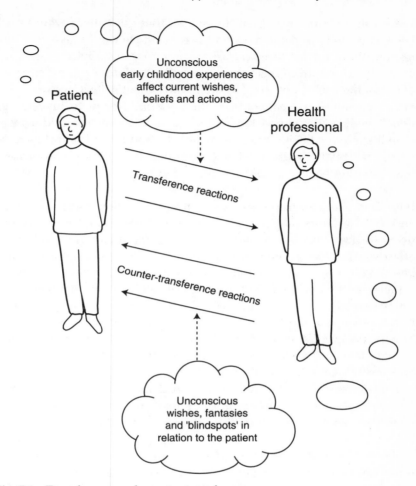

**Fig. 5.1** Transference and counter-transference.

*Clinical example*

Susan, a student nurse, found an adult male patient was making her the focus of his attention, telling her that she was his favourite nurse and eventually confiding that he had fallen in love with her. At first Susan ignored the disclosure and carried on nursing the patient as if the disclosure had not occurred.

'Working with the transference', however, meant that Susan was able to discuss this in a more open way with him. Gaining assistance from her mentor/supervisor, she felt more confident in being able to talk openly with the patient about these feelings and was able to explore the interactions more critically. Susan discovered that the patient would often behave in a very dependent way towards her. He would take very little responsibility for his care and ask her for constant advice. Susan was able to gently confront this behaviour and not collude with the situation of becoming such a powerful figure in the patient's life. Care was taken not to patronise the patient and not to be indifferent to his feelings, which were very real to him. This led to a more balanced way of working, so that Susan was able to feel she had better control over the situation. This is clearly a better way of dealing with such an incident than ignoring what was said – Susan's first way of dealing with it.

It is not unusual for patients to develop an infatuation towards the carer and such declarations can be very flattering! Some carers may even end up marrying ex-patients they have cared for. However part of the attraction is often related to transference, rather than being 'reality'-based. This is because the nature of the relationship between patient and carer is very unilateral. The carer does not usually share as much interpersonal or intimate information as the patient. During the course of the patient's admission he is asked to divulge a considerable amount of personal and intimate detail. This raises ethical considerations about 'power' within the relationship which demands that the carer does not take advantage of this position.

Transference reactions often occur in patients' relatives, who at times, in their powerlessness, often project unrealistic expectations on to the staff. This can be very seductive for the newly qualified carer, who may be tempted to give more information than she is sure about, in an attempt to be helpful. It is important that the carer is aware of this and offers only accurate information. When unsure of the reality, the carer can seek assistance from senior colleagues. It is important to feel able to say to patients or relatives, 'I don't know, but will find out for you'.

Not all transference reactions are positive. Very hostile reactions from patients are likely to be transference reactions. Early childhood responses to frustration, fear, or lack of control usually result in tantrums and verbal hostility towards parents. Such a response in adult life, while generally unacceptable, can be accounted for as unconscious 'replays' of childhood behaviour – for example the adult who 'sulks' after a request has been turned down, or who behaves in a childlike way as a reaction to frustration. The carer who is aware that this is happening will be able to deal more appropriately with the behaviour.

Counter-transference reactions can be equally powerful in affecting the interpersonal relationship. A typical counter-transference reaction may explain a very sudden or irrational dislike or attraction towards another person. Counter-transference occurs when previous experiences in the carer's life affect the carer's relationship with a patient. Consider the following example.

*Clinical example*

Martin, a student nurse, was working on ward 8, a medical care area. He was assigned to work with a middle-aged man who had been admitted with chest pains. Martin introduced himself to the patient, who seemed pleasant although anxious. However, Martin found himself disliking the patient. During the remainder of the day he found himself feeling irritated with the patient's questions and although he did not show these feelings, they were affecting his relationship with the patient.

On his way home from work that evening Martin felt guilty for being brusque with the patient on one occasion and wondered why he had felt irritated by this man, who had not behaved in any way to justify this reaction. He put this down to feeling tired and thought no more about it that day. Next day was his 'day off' and during the day he found himself thinking about his childhood, something he had not done for some time. His mother had divorced his father when Martin was young and later remarried. His stepfather was strict towards him and he recalled very unhappy memories of arguments between his mother and stepfather over how he was to be treated. Then it suddenly struck him that the patient he had cared for the previous day was very similar in appearance to his stepfather and also shared the same Christian name. This had not occurred to him at all during the previous day, but he now felt sure that this was why he had felt irritated and abrupt with him.

Now aware of the possible cause of his irritation, he was able to confront his feelings and rationalise his responses to this patient. He was able to respond more naturally and offer appropriate care.

This example gives a very clear indication of how powerful counter-transference reactions can be. The incident demonstrates how earlier unhappy memories, can be *repressed*, put 'out of mind', to re-emerge as powerful emotional responses in relation to another individual, the feelings being transferred.

Freud first described transference and counter-transference reactions when he noticed patients developed 'crushes' or infatuations for him. Feeling it unlikely that patients would find him attractive, he speculated how strong attachments might be due to the feelings being associated with earlier relationships in the patient's history. He argued that such feelings were likely to have resided as unconscious projections from previous associations and 'transferred' to the present time – a time of vulnerability for the patient. For the carer, observation and exploration of strong feeling is important in being able to respond appropriately. Understanding the dynamics helps identify more appropriate caring strategies.

Repression, as described earlier, is the mechanism whereby the anxiety is put out of awareness. In Chapter 2 an example was given of how repression can lead to the forgetting of very unpleasant occurrences. Many patients can only retain a very limited amount of information when anxious, due to the anxiety interfering with their attention span. This can act as a 'safety' mechanism, allowing a patient time to process what is happening to them. The carer has to take this into account when interacting with patients who are afraid, anxious or fearful, so that she does not overload the patient.

It is good practice not to give out too much information at once, repeating the important parts over a period of time. Carers, in a quest to appear helpful, may deluge newly admitted patients with information. Unfortunately this overburdens them with detail, most of which is not retained, or worse, can be misinterpreted. Information is better understood when paced at the patient's ability to take it in, rather than all at once.

Another common mechanism used by patients as a stress-relieving mechanism, is *regression*. This was introduced in Chapter 2, as a mechanism against anxiety, by reverting to an earlier period of development. It is a common mechanism and carers will often observe this in operation. Frequently patients will become giggly or seem to behave in very childlike ways, which can be very taxing for the carer, who cannot always see what the joke is about. It is often associated with dependent behaviour. When this occurs the patient will often try to attract attention at very frequent intervals. Patients become labelled as a nuisance or demanding and become 'unpopular' with the health care team. Consequently they become ignored by staff, and their anxiety gets worse, as they become cut off from constant reassurance.

Such behaviour is really masking unspoken or unacknowledged fear. Interpersonal skills, which can be applied by the carer to help the patient in such instances, begin with engaging the patient in conversation, taking care to listen to the possible areas of anxiety, identifying the possible cause, and reassuring the patient.

Offering reassurance is more of a process than a set of techniques. French (1983) describes reassurance as a means of restoring the patient's self-confidence. Loss of confidence in self or in the environment are common features of the anxiety patients feel when they become ill. Reassurance can be offered by being present and seeking to monitor the patient's progress. A study carried out in a coronary care unit found that patients were reassured when they felt the staff were monitoring their progress regularly, and appeared competent (Cronin and Harrison, 1988).

Carers can assist the patient by attempting to instil hope. When a person becomes ill, the stress of the illness becomes supported by the patient's ability to feel hopeful about the outcome. Hope requires information about the disease and awareness of progress (Sundeen *et al.*, 1994). Millar (1985) has suggested that 'hope' can be instilled in the following ways.

- Assisting the patient to maintain close relationships with their loved ones.
- Helping the patient to develop new coping skills.
- Allowing patients to regain as much control of their lives as possible.

The carer can work with the relatives and friends of the patient, encouraging them to assist and become involved in the care. It may be necessary to try to provide privacy for the relatives. Providing attention and information for the patient and relatives about what is happening helps to reduce anxiety and build hope.

Helping the patient to develop better coping skills and manage stress can be achieved by demonstrating basic relaxation skills, such as simple breathing exercises. Where the patient's breathing is affected by pain, it is clearly important that the patient is assisted by using appropriate analgesia. Deep breathing exercises are very much a part of basic care for non-ambulant patients. Therefore linking deep breathing exercises and encouraging the patient to relax muscles in the neck and shoulders, can be encouraged at regular intervals.

Massage is a very effective method of reducing stress and anxiety. After discussing this with the senior staff or supervisor, relatives can be encouraged to carry this out, and often only need encouragement or reassurance that it is perfectly in order. Where the patient is surrounded with technical apparatus such as tubing, drains or intravenous lines, the relatives can be shown how to access the patient appropriately, to enable gentle massage of head, neck or limbs.

*Clinical example*

Ms Jones, a 35-year-old, was admitted to the orthopaedic area after a motor bike accident where she fractured her left fibula and tibia (lower leg bones). On admission she was very anxious, declaring to the radiologist who was X-raying her that she was 'very afraid of hospitals.'

When she arrived at the ward she was prepared for the surgery. The surgical procedure was explained to Ms Jones by the surgical registrar, who went into careful detail to ensure that she was completely aware of what would happen. The nurse prepared her for the operation and noticed that she was very quiet. After leaving her for no more than two minutes while she checked the premedication chart, the nurse returned to find Ms Jones crying and clearly very distressed. It became clear from the subsequent discussion that she had not taken in any of the information the doctor had given her an hour earlier. The nurse carefully explained the operation, taking care to ensure Ms Jones understood what would happen to her. She was careful not to offer her facile reassurance and took her time to find out what her concerns were.

The nurse discovered that Ms Jones' partner had arrived and was waiting outside. She invited him in and explained the procedure again. The nurse also explained that Ms Jones' partner could stay with her while she was prepared for surgery. Ms Jones welcomed this and appeared more settled.

As well as the obvious consequences of shock due to the fluid loss, the effects of psychological shock must also be taken into account. For the caring team, who may unfortunately deal frequently with young adults in the aftermath of road traffic accidents, this may become almost routine. However, for the patient this is clearly a major catastrophic event.

Some patients do not wish their close relatives to see them upset. However, if carers work more closely with relatives and make the effort to interact and get to know them as well as possible, it may be easier to make suggestions that can be helpful. It is important to find out what the patients would like, so that if they prefer to be alone at times, this is respected. For many patients it is less stressful to have someone close to them at times of vulnerability and fear.

Other examples of defensive behaviour have been described by Satir (1972).

- Placating: Agreeing with everything that is said.
- Blaming: Defensive coping where the patient attempts to control the situation by diverting attention and fault to others.

- Computing: Rationalisation and attempts to 'intellectualise' fears and anxiety. Sometimes this can be exhibited as obsessive behaviour.
- Distracting: Ignoring perceived threat by focusing on irrelevant or apparently disconnected issues.

Such patterns of communication can often be seen in patients, who, for whatever reason, are anxious and avoid communicating their fears in more healthy ways. Alternatively, the defensive responses may be unconscious and therefore require the carer to attempt to uncover the anxiety. This may not be very easy to achieve at first attempt; defensive coping will be difficult to challenge and must be carried out gently. When the nature of the communication is 'defensive', it provides the carer with clues. The cause of the anxiety may be fairly obvious; however, if it is 'hidden' it will be necessary to develop the relationship further, establishing trust and reassuring the individual, gradually attempting to uncover the cause.

## Behavioural approaches

Behavioural approaches are based upon theories of learning which rely upon fundamental principles of reward or attention from others and reinforcement. The theoretical ideas are described in Chapter 2. This section will focus on how behavioural approaches can assist the health professional at a personal level, by examining assertiveness – a crucial interpersonal skill which enables the carer to interact with both the patient and other staff in a more effective way.

Learning to communicate in a direct and caring way, with consideration to both patient and carer, is referred to as *assertive communication*. Assertive behaviour skills have received much attention in the psychological literature (McCartan and Hargie, 1990). Non-assertive behaviours have adverse effects on the carer by creating stress and manipulative behaviour instead of direct and open communication (Bond, 1986) which may lead to lowered self-confidence, irritability and anger (McCartan and Hargie, 1990). Much of the discontent that health professionals feel has been attributed to the inability to express feelings appropriately, and to overpowering feelings of powerlessness, discontent and helplessness. If such feelings are present at work it is easy to understand why individuals leave their careers. In several nursing studies, morale and job satisfaction were considered to be severely affected by such feelings (Pardue, 1980).

Being able to interact effectively with patients and to act on their behalf requires carers who are able to be assertive (Webb, 1987). Assertiveness means communicating with others in a direct and honest way. The alternatives are to communicate aggressively, or at the other extreme, in a passive and submissive way. Communication can be considered as a continuum, with aggression at the extreme of one end, and passivity at the other (Fig. 5.2). Assertiveness is often defined as a way of interacting that attends to the needs of others, while at the same time regarding the *needs of self*. The carer can not meet the needs of everyone else, saying 'yes' to all demands. Assertiveness implies being able to say 'no', without feeling unduly guilty. This may be quite difficult for some carers. Health care is ostensibly about caring for others, which often creates the dilemma whereby carers find it impossible to say 'no' to demands for their attention. This eventually results in irritability and stress. Anger is the usual result, commonly taken out on partners, friends or members of family.

ASSERTIVE

Aggressive ◄————————————————————————————► Passive

| | |
|---|---|
| An aggressive approach may lead to physical or verbal violence. Aggressive behaviour frequently camouflages a basic lack of self-confidence, which leads to attempts to overpower others to 'prove' superiority. | The passive person consistently subordinates own rights to their perception of the rights of others. When angry, the passive person is thereby creating increased tension within himself. |

Assertiveness implies

Communicating one's feelings directly to others. This applies to both **positive** and **negative** feelings. As a result anger is not allowed to build up and the expression of feeling is more likely to be in proportion to the situation.

**Fig. 5.2**    Assertiveness – a continuum of behaviour.

Aggressive ways of interacting with others are often the result of a non-assertive interaction. Irritation with self, for allowing the situation to continue and feeling unable to confront the situation more openly, results in feeling persecuted by the demands, and irritable impulsive anger 'leaks' out. An extreme example of how serious this can become was in a couple where one of the partners was unable to say what her needs were. Feeling angry with her partner, but unable to express it, she would wreak revenge by cutting chunks out of her partner's collection of house plants while he was at work.

Saying 'yes' when the true response is 'no' is a sign of non-assertiveness. It is important to assess the reason for this failure. It has been noted earlier that many health care staff find it difficult to say no to others. Not being able to care for self, or give attention to one's own needs, can lead to eventual 'burn-out'. This is a stressful condition characterised by feelings of demotivation, disinterest, possible alcohol or tobacco abuse and unresolved anger. The sufferer loses satisfaction for their work. This is a tragic result of believing that it is impossible to allow personal needs to be respected. Passivity, or constantly agreeing to others' demands and needs, often leads to angry internal feelings. Assertiveness means listening in a genuine way to the needs of others, *while at the same time* taking into account personal needs and limitations.

Assertiveness is a behavioural skill that needs practice. For a personal assessment of assertiveness, the reader is invited to consider how many times during the past week 'yes' was given to a request, when the preferred, and more honest response was 'no!'. The essential skills of assertiveness are:

- self-awareness
- negotiation
- compromise
- calm insistence.

## *Self-awareness*

Self-awareness is an essential skill in *all* interpersonal interventions and one that requires continuous practice by the health professional. Burnard (1992) describes self-awareness as process of 'getting to know our feelings, attitudes, and values'. It is an ongoing process that can develop and mature each day. To be effective, the carer requires the skill of continuously self-appraising both herself and her work. This may sound a daunting task; however, the self-aware individual is better equipped to benefit from the ability to change, rather than remain stuck and institutionalised. Self-awareness and assertiveness require the carer to be honest and evaluate the ways in which she relates to others. This is the first step.

## Negotiation

Negotiating is a skill that improves with practice. The technique recognises the value of both personal needs and the needs of the other, and makes this explicit. Rehearsing the key points that are likely to arise in any anticipated intervention is very useful and, when negotiating, the carer has to be clear, what she is not prepared to give up.

## Compromise

Where it is difficult to reach agreement, the next best position is a working compromise. Again, the skill requires the carer to be aware of what 'ground' she is prepared to give up, so that she is reasonably content with the result. The technique aims to avoid the frustration and anger that is often the result of agreeing outwardly, then feeling compromised internally.

## Calm insistence

An important skill is to try to remain calm, even when the other party is being unreasonable. The technique is to state your position clearly and calmly, without anger, and then stick to it, repeating the point as necessary. Some texts refer to this skill as 'broken record' (Heron, 1973). The above skills can be practised and, like any skill, will improve. In common with learning any new skill, the techniques may also feel awkward and 'unrealistic' at first.

Behavioural approaches assert the importance of *reinforcement* as the means of encouraging desired behaviour. Reinforcement is achieved through rewarding appropriate behaviour. For most people, any human attention can be assumed to be rewarding in most instances, so that a smile, touch, confirmation that we have done well, all act as reinforcers.

Researchers have attempted to evaluate whether health professionals consider 'caring' behaviour in the same way that patients do. In research carried out with nurses and patients, Larson (1987) found a difference between how caring behaviours are perceived by each group. The study reported that nurses believed that 'comforting' and 'trusting' were most important, while patients considered 'accessibility' and 'following through' as being most important from their perspective. Behavioural approaches rely on accurate *assessment* and *planning*, therefore the above study indicates the importance of being clear that staff understand what behaviours the patient would consider as 'rewarding'. Also the significance of Larson's study for carers is the importance of ensuring accuracy about time and promises to 'be back in a few minutes'. For busy care staff a 'few minutes' may be an hour; however, for patients who are waiting, it may seem an eternity.

In summary, interpersonal skills based upon behavioural theory aim to identify a specific response or pattern of reactions by the patient and attempt to deal with this in as prompt a manner as possible. A prerequisite is the skill of learning to be assertive. This means caring in a way that attends to the needs of the patient (and of others around him), while at the same time being aware of one's own limitations. Assertiveness is the basic interpersonal skill of interacting in a realistic and more appropriate way. With practice it can become a way of surviving the inexhaustible demands of health care practice. Learning that taking care of *self needs* as well as the needs of others is not the same as being selfish. Doing so invariably leads to improved work satisfaction and a better tolerance to work stresses.

## Person-centred approaches

Long before the patient enters the hospital or the carer becomes professionally involved with the treatment prescribed, the patient will have made his own, tentative diagnosis (Oliver, 1993). The medical staff will attempt to make sense of the information provided and 'translate' this into medical terminology. So, for example, as Oliver suggests, 'a feeling of sickness' becomes 'nausea', and an accompanying feeling of 'tightness around the chest when I walked up the stairs' becomes a diagnosis of angina. The medical model conceptualises the patient's experience of his symptoms into a language that can only be communicated by another medical person. In other words communication consists of 'translations' between what the patient says, into terms which match the medical descriptions of disease in textbooks. This can effectively create a barrier between what the patient actually experiences and the health care staff who care for him.

In the opening account of this chapter, a patient describes graphically how he felt about the fact that many staff were unable to relate to him directly, as another person. Rather than deal with him, they related to the accompanying assortment of tubes and attachments. Other staff seemed, to him, to be too attached to the administrative aspects of his care – the rigour of collecting data and keeping accurate records. While these activities are without question important, fundamental interpersonal skills such as smiling and talking 'face to face' with him were often forgotten, or else overlooked by the care staff. This patient recalled a carer who he felt was more 'intuitive'. By this he meant a carer who seemed to *look, listen* and *attend* to his needs as a person, as well as caring medically. Person-centred care seeks to challenge the gap that can develop between these two positions by focusing more on the patient's experience.

Morse and Johnson (1991) suggest an alternative way of viewing illness to the more conventional 'medical model'. They consider illness behaviour as the ability of the patient to cope with or respond to the disease process. In this way, illness is viewed as consisting of an experience that affects the sick person and his immediate circle of family or friends. Interactions and roles that all individuals have hitherto developed are thrown into crisis and there is an attempt to compensate for the change. This approach to understanding illness may seem perplexing to many health workers who have been steeped in the conventional 'medical model' interpretation of what the patient says. Morse and Johnson (1991) describe this alternative view as the *illness constellation model*. The model has four stages:

- the stage of uncertainty
- the stage of disruption
- the stage of striving to regain self
- the stage of regaining well-being.

## The stage of uncertainty

This begins with the patient noticing changes that may indicate that something is wrong. The individual may confide in members of his family or may attempt to keep it to himself. Eventually, as the illness progresses, his family become aware that there are problems. For example a man in his early fifties noticed a lump in his chest. He was aware of the implications in women, but considered that men did not suffer from serious problems with their breasts. However the lump became painful and he consulted his doctor who referred him to a specialist. A biopsy was performed and he had to wait a week for the result.

Initially he kept the discovery of the lump to himself, but after the visit to his doctor, informed his wife. At that time he was more embarrassed about having to attend a 'clinic where he was the only man'. In this instance the news was good, the lump was diagnosed as 'benign'.

## The stage of disruption

This next stage is described by Morse and Johnson (1991) as a crisis point where the illness affects the well-being of the person who becomes ill and dependent upon the care staff. The patient copes with this by *distancing* himself from the situation. Friends and relatives are very affected by the patient's illness, which is often treated as if it were a threat to the stability of the family. In serious illness this is, of course, a reality.

## Striving to regain self

The next stage is the point in time when the patient is attempting to make sense of his illness. The patient may, for example, search his past for possible reasons for his illness, searching and striving for explanations and incidents which may have contributed to his situation. We all have a fundamental need to make sense of the world, and often, as health carers, do not give the patient sufficient time to explore these questions. There are seldom simple answers; however, allowing the patient to come to terms with his situation, by assisting him with this process, is very reassuring and comforting.

Loss and bereavement also create a search to make sense of what has happened. Accompanying the search is often self-recrimination, 'If only I did this', or 'I wish I had said this or done that'. Offering reassurance, by presenting reality in a gentle and calm way, for example providing the patient or relative with information about the illness, may assist understanding of the realities. This often assists the bereaved in being less judgemental about themselves.

## Regaining well-being

This final stage represents the overcoming of the illness. This may not mean achieving a permanent 'cure'. For patients with terminal illness, this stage may mean re-establishing most of the previous patterns of relationship with family and friends. The patient struggles with the issue of 'control' over his body and mind, and comes to achieve a more spiritual acceptance of what has occurred. The patient is able to 'take charge' and re-establish a renewed perspective.

The carer can help to confirm what is possible and allow the patient to gradually gain confidence in what they can achieve. Many illnesses have very successful outcomes, with a total return to a previously healthy status. However, following surgery or treatment, patients often rely on the staff to 'give permission' to carry out independent activity. Indeed, part of the carer's role is to encourage and maintain as much independence as possible. This requires confidence, which is why a trusting relationship is the foundation to helping patients recover.

Morse and Johnson (1991) suggest that the carer's role throughout all of the above stages is to *minimise suffering*. Suffering in this context needs to be conceived by examining the patient's experience in a holistic way. That is:

> '... both acute and chronic pain, the strain of trying to endure, the alienation of forced exclusion from everyday life, the shock of institutionalisation, and the uncertainty of anticipating the ramifications of the illness.'

> (Morse and Johnson, 1991)

Minimising suffering begins with the carer attempting to understand the patient's experience as he 'travels through' the stages. The specific interpersonal skill involved at this stage is to focus on what the patient actually says, or to encourage him to say more about his condition and how it affects him. Included with this is the importance of the opinions and views of those people around him. Family and friends can be asked how they feel he is progressing and for elaborations of how they perceive what is happening. Using the patient's own words rather than reclassifying them in medical terminology may help to build a more accurate picture of what is actually being experienced by the patient. This can inform carers about the most appropriate way of responding to his needs.

A person-centred approach has the *experiences of the patient* at the centre of any view of health or illness. Morse and Johnson suggest a move away from the disease-orientated, medical approach of ill health, using instead the assessment of needs and the *patient's* own experience, as a basis of understanding.

Kitson (1996) suggests that, in times of change to the provision of health care due to economic pressures, a valid question is whether the term 'caring' itself has any legitimacy. Today there is growing pressure for practice to be evidence-based and cost-effective. There is a danger of 'forgetting about the human being who also happens to be present with a treatable condition'.

Person-centred care begins by challenging the assumptions carers hold about their practice and beliefs about care, and suggests a revision –

a return to an understanding of the patient's beliefs and assumptions of their illness.

## Conclusions

In conclusion, the three approaches described in this chapter give differing views of how interpersonal responses can vary. The psychodynamic approach focuses on the significance of 'transference' reactions and the unconscious power of the carer–patient relationship. This view contends that awareness of this process is of fundamental importance to effective interpersonal skill. Behavioural skills rely more specifically upon the significance of assertiveness skills as important prerequisites to effective intervention.

Finally, the person-centred approach focuses more on the importance of what is going on in the present, with an attempt to understand the patient's total experience.

In reality, each of the above approaches may interact, and interpersonal skill consists of responding in the most effective way. What does unite any of these approaches can best be summed up by referring once again to the patient's view given at the beginning of this chapter. The interpersonally skilled carer is perhaps the individual who can learn to practise in such a way that she does not lose awareness of the importance of not only learning to be technically skilled, but also to continue to relate in an attending and sensitive way to the patient as a total human being.

## References

Bee, H. (1994) *Lifespan Development*. Harper Collins, New York.

Bond, M. (1986) *Stress and Self-awareness: A Guide for Nurses*. Heinemann, London.

Burnard, P. (1992) *Communicate: A Communication Skills Guide for Health Care Workers*. Edward Arnold, London.

Cronin, S.N. and Harrison, B. (1988) Importance of nursing care behaviours as perceived by patients after myocardial infarction. *Heart Lung* **17**, 374.

Erikson, E.H. (1980) *Identity and the Life Cycle*. Norton, New York.

French, P. (1983) *Social Skills for Nursing Practice*, 2nd edn. Chapman and Hall, London.

Heron, J. (1973) *Experiential training techniques*. Human Potential Research Project, University of Surrey, Guildford.

Holmes, J. and Lindley, R. (1991) *The Values of Psychotherapy*. Oxford University Press, Oxford.

Kessler, R.C., Foster, C., Webster, P.S. and House, J.S. (1992) The relationship between age and depressive symptoms in two national surveys. *Psychology and Ageing* 7, 119–26.

Kitson, A. (1996) A nurse's perspective. In *Essential Practice in Patient–centred Care* (K.W.M. Fulford, S. Ersser and T. Hope, eds). Blackwell Science, Oxford.

Larson, P.J. (1987) Comparison of cancer patients' and professional nurses' perceptions of important nurse caring behaviours. *Heart Lung* 16, 187.

McCartan, P.J. and Hargie, O.D.W. (1990) Assessing assertive behaviour in student nurses: a comparison of assertive measures. *Journal of Advanced Nursing* 15, 1370–76.

Millar, J.F. (1985) Inspiring hope. *American Journal of Nursing* 85, 23.

Morse, J.M. and Johnson J.L. (1991) *The Illness Experience: Dimensions of Suffering.* Sage Publications, London.

Oliver, R.W. (1993) *Psychology and Health Care.* Bailliere Tindall, London.

Pardue, S.F. (1980) Assertiveness for nursing. *Supervisor Nurse* 11(2), 47–50.

Rindfuss, R.R. (1991) The young adult years: diversity, structural change and fertility. *Demography* 28, 493–512.

Satir, V. (1972) *Peoplemaking.* Science & Behaviour Books, Palo Alto, California.

Sundeen, S.J., Stuart, G.W., Rankin, E.A.D. and Cohen, S.A. (1994) *Nurse–Client Interaction*, 5th edn. Mosby, St Louis, Missouri.

Webb, C. (1987) Speaking up for advocacy. *Nursing Times* 83(34), 33.

# Further reading

Fulford, K.W.M., Ersser, S. and Hope, T. (eds) (1996) *Essential Practice in Patient-centred Care.* Blackwell Science, Oxford.

# Chapter 6
# Approaches to the Care of the Older Patient

This chapter will explore the influences of the three theoretical approaches – psychodynamic, behavioural and person-centred, in relation to the older patient. The section begins with a general discussion of ageing, and sets the context for the three ways of looking at the person who becomes unwell. As with previous chapters, it begins with an account from a carer, in this case a junior medical student, which may capture many of the preconceived views about the older patient that health carers bring into practice with them.

*Jane – third year medical student*

'I suppose I held all the usual prejudices about working with old people, possibly by having to study the disorders in the elderly as part of my course. So I tended to expect every person to be either deaf or dementing at first, which was incredibly crass! Having been brought up as a child with memories of staying at my grandparents, I can remember them putting their teeth into pots to soak overnight in the bathroom. I can recall being fascinated by the shape of the pink palate and rows of white teeth, magnified in the glass. My parents impressed on me the importance of brushing my teeth regularly and I used to think how horrible it must be to have a removable mouth. Nowadays, due to better dental health care and improved diet, when I reach old age I am likely to have very good teeth. So in my later years my own grandchildren are unlikely to be treated to seeing my teeth chattering on the bathroom shelf!

I am aware of the striking demographic changes which have occurred over the past few decades, with the percentage of the elderly population steadily growing and life expectancy increasing. I see this in my work every day and it does create clinical dilemmas, for example, about how long to keep treating an elderly person with a chest infection with antibiotics, and when this is 'interfering with nature'.

At first I was hesitant when interacting with older patients. I felt they saw me as being very young and would often comment about this. Sometimes I imagined it was due to a fear on their part of having inexperienced practitioners caring for them. Some individuals would be very 'nice' about it and compliment me on looking very young while entrusting me completely with their treatment. Other patients were actually hostile and made it very clear that they 'did not want someone just out of school to look after them'. This was quite hurtful, particularly when I was unable to get much help from the team I was assigned to. Senior colleagues would just laugh when I reported back to them and told me to 'be more tactful'. Thinking back, I think I was very defensive. I would go back to face the patient, trying to be reassuring, but never really felt very comfortable and ended up making matters worse. Physical examinations of some patients was particularly fraught. There was often considerable embarrassment for both of us. This tended to make me even more self-conscious and caused me to fumble. Gradually, however, I think I managed to relax and feel less defensive, able to listen closely and more carefully to what they were telling me. This enabled me to deal more effectively with their worries and concerns, and my confidence grew. I think I was then less patronising because I was less anxious myself.

I now enjoy working with this client group. I was fortunate to have a very good relationship with my grandparents, one of whom died a few years ago. I think this has affected me. I find myself identifying with some of my patients when they remind me of them, particularly my grandad who died. This can be very upsetting for me sometimes when I feel myself getting involved with a family who have an elderly relative who is dying. I find that I can get 'too close' to these feelings but of course have to remember that the family is expecting me to be calm and in control.

I feel that working in health care settings can create a distorted perspective of the older person's health. This is due to working constantly with the crisis periods of health in this population. Working with a number of confused elderly people during one particularly busy shift, I remember stopping at the traffic lights on my way home to let two very elderly people cross. It suddenly struck me that there are more healthy elderly people 'out there' who are coping very well and enjoying reasonably good health. I now find working with the elderly a very rich source of stimulation and challenges, both clinically and personally. Time permitting, I do enjoy the conversation and the relationships which build up with this client group. Generally, they are more open and relaxed'.

In the above account, Jane made reference to the steadily increasing number of people over the age of 65 years of age. This change is likely to continue to grow, reaching a peak in 2040 (Bee, 1994; Fig. 6.1). It is not surprising that the study of ageing and gerontology, the scientific study of the conditions affecting the older patient, has become more popular during the past decade. In 1900 only 1 person in 30 was over 65. By 1970 this had increased to one person in nine, and by the year 2020 it is likely to be one person in five over the age of 65 years (Eisdorfer, 1983). The effects of this increase will obviously have significant effects upon the Health Service and, indeed, the culture of every country affected.

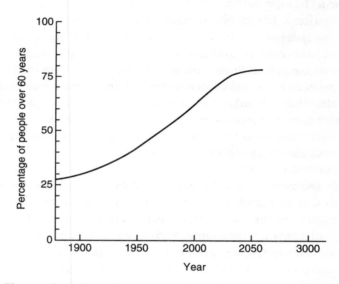

**Fig. 6.1**   The number of people over the age of 65 years will continue to grow, reaching a peak in the year 2040.

Within families, there will be more pressure to care for ageing relatives. As the health and general well-being of this group also improves, a number of positive benefits in terms of families having grand- and great-grandparents alive will occur, in many cases sharing the upbringing of children. An increase in health care costs will develop, with greater demand for housing, pension plans and welfare payments. Every part of society is likely to become affected by these changes. The growing number of fit and healthy elderly are likely to gain more political power as this group gains an increasing share of the vote. Television advertisements will also reflect the larger viewing numbers of this group; perhaps 'Levi 501s' will become targeted at the 50-plus age group!

# Health and the elderly

Publication of the government White Paper in the UK, *The Health of the Nation* (1992), has raised a number of important questions concerning the health of older people and has set targets for health workers. For example, numerous targets have been set in relation to cancer screening, incontinence, prevention of osteoporosis, strokes, depression, dementia, accidents, respiratory diseases and health promotion. Also targets for the support of lay carers is mentioned. The list is extensive and has been criticised for failing to give sufficient space to promoting prevention of illness (McDermott, 1995).

Age Concern (1992) has argued that rehabilitation is so vital in promoting independence that it merits being a key area for increased resources. Henwood (1992) has suggested that health workers' attitudes and knowledge about ageing become, in themselves, severe barriers to providing correct support to the elderly. Like Jane's honest disclosure about attitudes towards the elderly, there is much ignorance and inaccurate generalisation about ageing. For her, the reality of actually working with this group of people allowed her to reassess her prejudice. Many health workers unfortunately do not.

Respect for the old is certainly a function of the political and cultural traditions of a society. The views of the older person may be rejected as old-fashioned, simply because they come from an aged body (Raynor, 1986). Retirement creates a place for a member of the younger generation to step into, and society sets a compulsory retirement age. At the time of writing, the UK Government is considering changes to the current national retirement age of 60 years for women and 65 years for men.

The generic phrase 'elderly' or 'older person' does not help to clarify attitudes towards being old. A fairly crude but nevertheless widely-used subgrouping has been used in America. This is to divide the elderly into the *young old* and the *old old*. (Neugarten, 1974, 1975 in Bee, 1994). The 'young old' are those between 55 and 75 years and the 'old old' those people over 75 years. The two categories are used to differentiate the risks to health or the occurrence of illness. The importance of this division is the classification of age group associated with particular health problems. Clearly, the risk of more serious ill health is in the group over the age of 75, where there is likely to be a decline in hearing ability and mobility. Research over the past few decades has, however, demonstrated that the process of ageing varies with each individual, so the health worker really needs to take care in making generalised assumptions related to age – a fact discovered by Jane in the opening account of this chapter.

## Psychodynamic considerations

Erikson (1959) claimed that the key task in old age is to resolve a personal crisis which he called *integrity versus despair*. A sense of integrity, according to Erikson, was the ability to develop a sense of living a meaningful life and an acceptance of the process of ageing. This does not mean a passive existence and then decline. Rather, it refers to a new appraised sense of purpose and fulfilment through acceptance of the realities of ageing: being able to reflect on a 'life review', considering both the happy and successful accomplishments with an acceptance of the disappointments and sadness; then to develop further, with energy, new projects which are achievable within individual personal limits. The ability to reflect on a review of life and to reminisce, was for Erikson a crucial part of satisfactory adjustment in old age.

The clinical significance of this idea has been incorporated into various interpersonal approaches in the care of the older person. *Reminiscence therapy* is practised in many areas and consists of encouraging the recall of past events and allowing the older patient to describe their past. Until the 1960s this was considered to be a harmful activity for older people as it was thought to encourage 'living in the past' (Olds, 1995). Today, however, a better understanding of the positive effects of reminiscence has become integrated into practice (Rimmer, 1982).

One method is to organise a group of people to sit around in a circle so that they can easily see and hear one another. The room should be free of noise and interruptions. The health worker 'leads' the discussion and a choice of 'themes' can be helpful. Examples would be choosing topics like 'seaside holidays', or may be simply encouraging each person to recall memories from childhood. Because long-term memory is not so affected by disorders of memory, most older people will have rich memories to share. As in all groups the members will require encouragement to join in. The occasions are often best when arranged informally, say around an afternoon tea break. However, the skill of leading sessions is in creating a relaxed atmosphere, perhaps with the health worker leading with personal accounts, to get things going. Comparing events from the past with the present helps to orientate the person who is confused. For example, comparing the prices of everyday items, such as the price of a loaf of bread or pint of milk, helps to orientate the person in the present.

Developmentally, old age, like adolescence, is also a time of fairly rapid change. For example, retirement brings a sudden change of self-identity. In contemporary society, the daily routine of working life gives a sense of security. Despite the increasing number of people who are unable to find employment, earning a satisfactory wage continues as a main yardstick of relative success in life. Despite more education about preparing for retirement, the actual change often creates profound uncertainty and difficulties in adjusting to the new lifestyle for many people. For such individuals there is an intellectual preparation and understanding of what the change may produce; however, emotionally, the abrupt change in status is upsetting. It often creates vacillating periods of depression which are connected with the 'loss' of identity, status and power. This may produce angry responses, as an internal defence against these feelings. The anger is often projected on to those closest; so spouse, children and relatives will notice the difference and complain about the individual seemingly changing from being generally relaxed and confident, to becoming tense, irritable and belligerent.

Any period of change is stressful and bouts of physical illness may accompany this transition time. It is at this time that health workers may have contact with the patient and, because of the internalised anger, may also become unwitting recipients of this projected anger. Such anger may account for the irritation that Jane described at the beginning of this chapter, where some patients were hostile for having such a 'young' person taking care of their needs.

Loss of any description is nearly always accompanied by anger. It can be inanimate, such as loss of a purse or wallet, or loss associated with living. The poet Philip Larkin writes about, the loss of losing his hair in midlife 'not a crushing loss, but nevertheless a loss'. Loss of job and all the attendant feelings always requires considerable readjust-ment. Anger, rage and paranoid reactions are not uncommon. Loss is always accompanied by a period of *mourning*. Eventually the negative feelings are replaced by more satisfying substitutes. The health worker can play an important role in assisting with this natural transition. The basic skills are to firstly be aware of where the anger may be coming from, rather than taking it personally. It is not easy to remain non-defensive when someone is being hostile or rude. Like Jane in her account, becoming defensive seems to occur as an automatic response. The skill is to attend carefully to what is being said and to listen for the true message; that is, to ask oneself what may be behind the anger and attempt to address this. It may not work very well. Consider the following example.

*Clinical example*

Mrs Holt is a 67-year-old woman who had until recently worked in the reception area of the local community hospital. That was until 6 months ago when she retired from this work. Today, she was attending outpatients for investigations for possible stones in the biliary tract (gall stones). The history suggested intermittent pain, which, while not serious, had caused discomfort, particularly after a heavy meal. Mrs Holt was a proud and intelligent woman who was well aware of the medical implications of her symptoms.

On arrival she was greeted by Amanda, a first-year student nurse who was on a short placement in the department. Mrs Holt was surprised that nurses 'were allowed to train at such a young age' and proceeded to react angrily to Amanda's attempt to document her recent history. Mrs Holt felt questions about her dietary habits were her 'own business' and 'anyway I have already gone into all of this with my family doctor' who she 'had known for over 20 years!'. Mrs Holt did not see the point of relating all of this to someone so junior and asked to see 'someone of more senior rank'. Amanda attempted to explain that she was a student and had to learn, but felt herself angry and upset and remonstrated that she was not 'just out of school' and had been a student nurse for over 6 months. This escalated rather than abated the antagonism, and the interaction failed.

Examination of this account reveals how Amanda failed to pick up vital cues which may have helped to avoid the defensive opening of this dialogue.

First, she was aware that, until her recent retirement, Mrs Holt had been working as a hospital receptionist. While this is not a definite signal that Amanda will meet hostility to her questions, it is possible to develop skill and sensitivity when situations become fraught. At the first sign of an angry response, Amanda could have paused, reflecting on what *may* be behind the anger or discontent, rather than reacting to it. Checking the person's past and their lives and the context in which the illness has occurred, can often provide vital information beforehand.

An awareness of the psychodynamic mechanisms of **displacement** (see Chapter 2) enable the health worker to think about possible explanations other than this being simply an 'angry irritable patient'. There is a tendency to unconsciously 'transfer' the feelings of loss and anger on to others as a means of trying to deal with them. This process involves a form of temporary envy of others who still have their routines and the status their work brings them. For the individual who is in the transitional phase of attempting to deal with their own retirement, these feelings can become excessive and be projected on to others. Such bitterness is often only a temporary feeling, and indeed some older people who are better able to confront their true feelings, never experience a sense of bitterness. They are able to adapt in a more healthy way. So in this instance there was information that may have alerted Amanda. Mrs Holt had recently retired and from a job where she was regularly dealing with medical and health staff and 'patients'. Having to assume the opposite role is often difficult for people who have worked in the health service!

### Health promotion in old age

Carl Jung, the Swiss analytic psychologist, was more interested in the second half of life. He felt that the first part of life was concerned with growing up, finding a partner and having a family; therefore moving into mid and later life requires a reappraisal and planning for the future. Jung felt that the earlier dreams of youth are put 'on-hold' for most individuals during the hectic family-rearing period. It is therefore necessary to encourage the older person to think about what they would like to achieve once these tasks have become fulfilled and there is potentially more free time.

Individuals who manage to keep an internal 'childlike' enthusiasm for new experiences tend to do better in old age. Raynor (1986) argues that a sense of purpose and contentment in old age also comes from a feeling of being able to continue to contribute to the welfare of others.

Argyle et al. (1989) have researched the concept of 'happiness', and factors such as remaining in contact with other people and interacting with others are identified as being very important. For the patient with a longer-term chronic illness, it is not only the debilitating physical and psychological effects of the actual condition, but also the sense of isolation which is a factor of prolonged ill health. Where this occurs, health workers can take action to encourage as much interaction as possible. This will obviously be limited by the patient's condition; however, where possible, activities can be planned and carried out. For instance, activities involving groups of patients of similar age can be encouraged, and carers can stress the importance of regular visits from friends and members of the family.

At the age of 84, Erikson published the results of a long-term study of people in their eighties (Erikson *et al.*, 1986). He had been collecting data on this group since 1928. In his book Erikson describes a prescription for achieving satisfaction and 'ego integrity' in later life. He argues that the older person must maintain active involvement in the world around him, rather than give up at retirement. They must, he argued, 'retain active participation and seek challenges and stimulation from those around them', developing new skills and interests. Health workers can play an active part in facilitating patients to reconsider their lifestyles as they recover from, or seek to cope with, debilitating illness.

The consideration of applied interpersonal skills within this approach is very much linked to Erikson's concept of 'integrity versus despair'. Thus the main aim is to maintain the patient's integrity as much as possible while avoiding becoming patronising. In many older people there is a gradual awareness of declining ability, or else an anxiety that this is occurring. Thus the patient who has periods of forgetfulness may maintain a pretence in order to avoid the embarrassment they may cause. In extreme situations this is described as 'confabulation', where the patient may 'invent' parts of an account in order to give the impression of integrity. When this occurs the carer is required to understand that this can become an unconscious mechanism, which also gives the patient 'internal reassurance', rather than being a deliberate deception. Carers can be very reassuring by offering ways of minimising the anxiety. For example, when it becomes apparent that a patient is unable to retain information about what is happening, the carer can take care to ensure that information is broken down into smaller parts which are repeated more often.

As admission to hospital or the effects of illness itself can be very disorientating, the carer has an important role to play in reducing the patient's anxiety through constant re-orientation. Close and constant observation is essential in such situations, and the care team will need to plan this as effectively as possible while maintaining the individual's dignity.

## Behavioural approaches in old age

The behavioural approach with its stress on learning is not often thought to be a suitable interpersonal approach to use in the elderly. This is due to concerns about the gradual decline in memory. It is very questionable from an ethical as well as clinical position, whether to use techniques which include an expectation of learning from reinforcing desired behaviour in such conditions. However, the maxim 'you can't teach an old dog new tricks' has to be treated with caution! There is now an extensive body of research that shows that with appropriate training older adults can significantly improve their performance in a variety of areas. For example, older people can improve their ratings on memory and intelligence tests, and can maintain this improvement over a long period of time (Kliegl *et al.*, 1989; Willis and Nesselroade, 1990; Verhaeghen *et al.*, 1992). Thus the impact of behaviour-based approaches is still very relevant with this age group. The term mental *plasticity* is often used to refer to a theoretical view that the developmental changes in life are very much a product of how frequently an individual 'exercises' their mind, as well as the effects of heredity and other physiological factors. There is some evidence that constant use of intellectual activities such as reading, discussion and mental reasoning can improve mental functioning (Busse and Wang, 1971).

Often the procedure of admitting older patients into hospital can precipitate confusion and anxiety, so that there is more forgetfulness, which in turn creates even more anxiety and greater memory inter-ference. This can increase at night, when there is less visual orientation for the person. Simply keeping the patient's night-light on throughout the night can be tried, and may help to alleviate some fear caused by 'disorientation'. Constant reinforcement and reassurance can help to settle such fear and help to break this cycle. A brief behavioural plan of explaining and repeating the explanation, while at the same time rewarding the patient through encouragement and praise, can be implemented as a way to deal with temporary confusion in a newly-admitted patient.

A form of therapeutic approach which seeks to correct disorientated speech in the elderly has been developed by Naomi Feil (1982). This approach is called *validation therapy* and was developed by Feil over a 20-year period. It is a reaction against the so-called *reality orientation methods* which have been developed to help confused and dementing patients. (Reality orientation is described in the following section.) According to Feil, some patients are unable to cope with the painful and present reality and so retreat to an 'inner reality' based on feelings rather than intellect. The patient with dementia retreats to the past to avoid stress, boredom and loneliness in the present. Validation therapy seeks to correct this retreat, by acknowledging the emotion and feelings expressed by the patient while at the same time confronting the disorientation. This is then rewarded and behaviour improves.

There is some recent research to suggest this may be an effective method (Bleathman and Morton, 1992). However, the approach is not without its critics. For example, Goudie and Stokes (1989) have suggested that confused messages from the client are attempts to make sense of what is happening to them at that moment in time and does not necessarily indicate confabulation.

Behavioural approaches thus have an important contribution to make in the care of the older patient. Any method whereby the carer attempts to use a 'reward' of some kind, such as a comment, 'You are doing very well Mr Jones ... well done', or even a smile, is a form of behavioural approach which seeks to increase the desired behaviour. However, it can only be argued to be an 'interpersonal approach' when it is implemented as part of a care plan.

## Person-centred approaches in the elderly

The focus of this approach is assessment of *needs* and the ability of the health worker to allow the patient freedom to participate in self-care. One of the founders of this approach, Abraham Maslow, studied a number of people from history whom he described as '*self-actualisers*', that is, capable of maintaining a quest for growth and development. Many of the subjects he considered as self-actualisers were well into their sixties and were still motivated towards reaching their potential.

For Jane at the beginning of this chapter, working with the elderly was a stimulating activity, partly because she found older people were able to relate in a more open way. Many people, as they get older, find that they are not as affected by the need to impress or the 'vanity of youth' which often interferes with the ability to relax in the company of others when we are younger. The older person who has accepted his position in life with calmness is often perceived as wise and understanding. Wisdom is a difficult concept to analyse; however, it may be that there is an accumulation of insight, knowledge and experience of life that endows some older people with sound judgement and the ability to counsel others (Sternberg, 1990).

The person-centred approach is fundamentally based in the 'here- and now', where skills are associated with the current needs of the person. The importance of listening to any patient in an attentive way can never be emphasised enough and is clearly a fundamental interpersonal skill.

The carer has to listen and understand the message being communicated, particularly when the patient is confused or disorientated. Deficit in visual acuity and hearing often worsens with age, therefore it may be best to sit directly facing a person who is deaf, so that the patient who has learnt to partially lip-read can do so. When interviewing or just talking, sitting where eye contact can be maintained with relative ease, and fairly close to others, facilitates communication.

Most sitting-rooms in elderly care areas are often arranged to suit the institution rather than aid interaction between patients. The writer can recall an experiment he carried out in an elderly assessment ward. The chairs in the unit were mainly arranged in straight rows; magazines were on shelves which were either difficult for the patients to access, or were out of date. Moving the chairs into small circular groups, ensuring that patients could thus see each other and were closer together so that they could hear one another, led to a dramatic improvement in communication and increased conversation between patients (Fig. 6.2). Asking staff to bring in more recent magazines rather than the five-year-old copies of *Homes and Gardens* which tend to clutter many waiting room areas, also assisted in helping to orientate patients in the 'here and now'.

A number of specific techniques have been developed to improve interpersonal communication. ***Reality orientation*** is the skill of giving patients constant information about their environment in a structured and systematic way. The aim is to encourage independence. Reality orientation (RO) was first used in the care of the elderly in the 1960s. Olds (1995) describes several forms of this approach, however, the most relevant in this context is the '24-hour' or 'informal reality orientation'. Twenty-four-hour RO is performed throughout the day and when necessary during the night. The patient is reminded of the day, date, season and time of day, at regular intervals. This is a team approach involving all staff with the aim of orientating the patient at all times so that he is aware of where he is and what is happening to him. When used at night, the method refers to dealing with the confused patient, offering reassurance by orientating in 'time and place'.

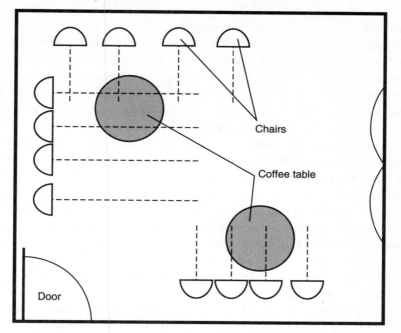

(a) Plan of Sitting Room-before

Chairs

Coffee table

Door

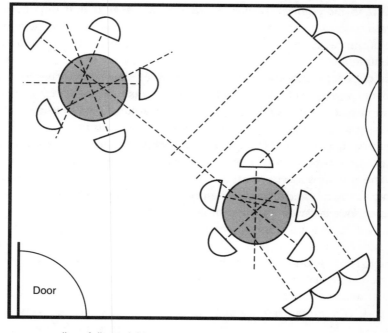

(b) Plan of Sitting Room-afterwards

Door

------ line of direct sight

**Fig. 6.2** Rearrangement of a sitting room to aid communication between patients.

Another technique is *resolution therapy*. This is an attempt to find the 'hidden meaning' within the confused speech. It is an individualised method of attending to the emotional element of speech, rather than the 'content'. Olds (1995) uses the example of the elderly confused patient who repeatedly pleads to be 'allowed home to look after her children who have just come home from school'. Rather than humouring the person, such as informing her that her 'children have in fact grown up', or giving ineffectual reassurance, this approach seeks to uncover the nature of the anxiety beneath the surface. Olds argues that the patient's confused request may be an attempt to communicate 'a fear of entrapment' (Olds, 1995). This is a feeling of being disempowered, a childlike feeling of being trapped. By showing empathetic concern and understanding, and not facile reassurance, feelings of security and trust can be enhanced. Then the health worker can help to reassure the patient that the children are not at risk of danger or harm.

So far in this chapter the approaches have been concerned primarily with the confused or dementing older patient. There are, however, a number of specific issues that affect the older person and become a source of major anxiety. For many people there is a real fear of increasing dependency and of becoming a burden to those around them. We all value our independence, perhaps without even thinking much about it, until it is threatened. Connected to this is a fear that if dependency increases, the security of knowing whether there will be someone to take care of our needs becomes a growing worry and leads to a cycle of fear and depression.

Helplessness, or fear of being helpless, is another possible cause of the kind of angry reactions that Jane experienced in her account at the beginning of this chapter. Thus the health worker may not immediately understand the anger displayed by the patient, who may be making a good physical recovery from illness. It is therefore helpful to explore the patient's perception of illness and their ideas and fears about recovery, particularly after leaving hospital. The patient may have concerns about being alone, or of putting more pressure on close relatives or a frail partner. When this is found to be the case, reassurance can be given by the health care team through good patient education and explanation of the services that may be available to assist both the patient and his family. There is often little individual knowledge, or family awareness, of what is available to help the patient live at home.

Examination of Maslow's 'hierarchy of needs' (see Chapter 2) suggests the human requirement for security and safety is a very basic one. Many elderly people entertain fears about growing incapacity and an inability to remain independent. These fears can be tackled in a direct and supportive way, encouraging the patient to be able to express the anger and helplessness, remembering that when this does begin to happen, it is tempting to interrupt, to offer reassurance. However, at first it may be sufficient and more therapeutic to simply listen and give acknowledgement to what is voiced. There are no 'rights or wrongs' in this context, and if the carer feels the patient is seeking verbal reassurance then it is certainly appropriate to do so. However, when the attempts at giving reassurance are reacted to with indifference, or even more anger and withdrawal, it is better to not say anything. 'Being present', remaining calm and giving acknowledgement to what is being said, rather than jumping in with well-intentioned but trite comment, is usually more helpful. It is important for everyone to feel that concerns have been heard and understood.

## Depression and suicide risk

Depression is a very common feature in later life, with high rates of suicide occurring in older men. The health care worker will frequently have to deal with the patient who presents with an underlying clinical depression. Being aware of the possible manifestations is important. The patient's history is the first consideration. Where there is a history of depressive reactions, or even previous attempts at suicide, the risk of such patients making further attempts must be considered as high. This is compounded where there is a current chronic health concern. The level of interaction the individual has with family, and socially, is another factor. When there is little social integration in the patient's life, with little or no social contact, the risk may be higher.

Sleep disturbances usually accompany depressive reactions. In the elderly, the pattern of sleep often changes anyway. The older person usually enters a lighter sleep and may take regular 'cat-naps'; thus there may be less need for the full 'eight hours' required in the past. In clinical depression, early morning wakening, that is waking at three or four o'clock in the morning after an agitated and restless night's sleep, is a common pattern. The person then finds it impossible to get back to sleep and feels nothing but gloom and blackness.

Appetite is usually reduced in the elderly and in depression may be practically absent. There is a need to ensure the patient remains hydrated, as the motivation to drink or take any nourishment may be totally absent in more extreme cases of depression, so regular drinks can be encouraged, such as small amounts of fruit juice.

## Close observation

Constant observation may be necessary, particularly when the patient is mobile and can get to the bathroom. If he is considered to be high risk, the patient may need to be supervised during a bath. Observation should be as unobtrusive as possible, while ensuring that the patient is safe and the health worker is aware of what he is doing at all times. Maintaining privacy within these limitations is often very difficult. It may be necessary to discuss the reasons for the intrusion in an open and honest way with the patient, rather than creep around in an unsuccessful attempt to be invisible!

It is also very important to observe for other signs of suicidal intent, such as hoarding prescribed medication. When suicidal intent has been mentioned by the patient or even if it is suspected by the staff, it needs to be raised and discussed with the patient. Many health workers avoid this, fearing the possibility of making the situation worse or of embarrassing the patient. The reality is that where suicidal feelings are present, talking openly with the patient will not 'put further ideas' into the person's mind. If there is a clinical depression with suicidal risks, the ideas will be there anyway. Attempting to accurately assess feelings and summon early and appropriate help from the psychiatric services may help to reduce the patient's suffering. The patient may also feel less isolated through the concern shown to him. All too often there exists a collusion of silence around those suffering with depression. Much of this may come from the health worker's own fears about dealing with the patient's condition.

### Clinical example

Mr Jenkins was a 69-year-old man admitted in a confused and disorientated state of mind. He was severely dehydrated and malnourished. Both the police and his doctor were involved after calls from his neighbours who had been concerned that they had not seen him for several days. He was treated with intravenous fluids and antibiotic medication, as he had developed a chest infection. His wife had died from heart failure 6 months before and he now lived alone after 40 years of married life. He had a son who was now living in Australia. His elder brother had died a year ago.

After two days in hospital he began to recover, although he was withdrawn and appeared to be clinically depressed. He told the staff that he 'didn't want to go on living ... and just wanted to be left alone to die'. The staff were concerned about his condition; however, their emphasis was on his physical condition. On one occasion a nurse discovered that he was not taking his antibiotics and that after they were dispensed to him he kept them in his mouth until the staff had moved on. He then collected them in an envelope he kept in his bedside locker. At first it was thought that he was not taking them to prevent the treatment from clearing up his condition, but later he confided that he was 'storing them up to take all at once'. He had wanted to anaesthetise his emotional pain and end his suffering.

A psychiatric referral was made and he was assessed as a suicidal risk. He was prescribed anti-depressant medication and seen regularly by the psychiatric services. His care consisted of very close observation and supervision and he gradually improved. He was discharged home with social and psychiatric follow-up, and attended a day hospital one day a week. Sadly, he died 6 months later of a chest infection, following a severe bout of influenza. The care team had tried to attend to his care, however they were convinced that he had 'given up' and offered little or no resistance to the infection.

Although tragic, this account emphasises how morale and motivation are important in the outcome of a person's illness. Mr Jenkins, despite the offers of help, did not want to go on living after his wife had died. However, staff can do much to encourage the patient and it is necessary to feel able to address the issues openly and directly with patients who seem to have lost hope. In many other cases it is possible to motivate the person to carry on and adapt to the loss. It is necessary to encourage the expression of grief and to allow the patient to articulate the meaning of their loss and feel supported by those around them. Sadly, it is the isolated and lonely person who is most at risk.

## Dealing with death and dying

The health worker will have to confront patients who are dying and help patients and their relatives come to terms with this. Personal awareness and attitudes to death and dying will play a significant part in how they are able to develop skills in this important area. Many health workers may not have had to deal with this issue within their own sphere of experience. Having to care for the dying or handling a death may therefore be a source of some fear. It is important to be personally honest and discuss these feelings with a trusted friend or colleague. It is always a good process to work alongside a more experienced member of staff when having to deal with this for the first time, which is often the practice. However, it is better to be open and feel able to express fear or concerns. Apprehension about the unknown is very natural and experienced by all staff at first.

After dealing with a death, it is important to make time with colleagues to review what has happened and again to express feelings about the incident. Being open and honest is helpful if upset. Gradually, confidence develops and the carer will be able to adopt a healthy approach to dealing with such situations. Even experienced staff are upset by the deaths of patients in their care, which is a healthy sign. It is much more acceptable within health care practice today to be able to admit to such fears and concerns, than perhaps it was in the past.

# Conclusions

For the majority of elderly people, and a continually growing number, there are more choices available in old age than existed in the past. The world has become a smaller place. Keeping contact with family and friends is cheaper and easier to do. An increasing number of older people are able to choose when to retire, how they would like to spend their time and where they would like to live. All of these choices can mean greater freedom and more independence. However, choice is constrained by health. Among individuals aged between 60 and 67 years, poor health raises the probability of early retirement by up to 20% (Sammartino, 1987).

Health can be improved through adopting a healthier lifestyle and health care workers can be effective in promoting good health in this age group. There is evidence that exercise is a very important variable which has been associated with longevity and also a greater feeling of well-being. Studies have also demonstrated that exercise improves physical functioning, such as physical flexibility, balance and reaction times (Rikli and Busch, 1986). Gentle and regular exercise routines can be undertaken by the majority of elderly and can be encouraged by health staff. Attention to a well-balanced diet, which includes low fat, high vitamin and sufficient protein, also contributes to healthiness. A diet rich in fibre can also prevent constipation and possible bowel complications in later life.

Emotional security is often closely associated with interpersonal relationships. As can be seen from the previous case example, Mr Jenkins gave up wanting to live after his wife had died. Research suggests that relationships in later life create higher satisfaction than in early life. However this satisfaction is of a different nature, based less on 'passion' and more on loyalty, familiarity and mutual investment within the relationship (Bee, 1994).

Relationships in later life seem to be better when partners see each other as a trusted means of support, as 'best friends' as well as partners, and where there is 'playfulness' and humour (Laurer and Laurer, 1985).

It is also the case that sexual activity does not cease after a certain age! Health carers must also become more concerned with addressing concerns that patients have about their sexual lives. Sexual relationships are an important part of all life, and yet there is often another embarrassed silence in health care settings when it comes to offering advice to recovering patients or generally dealing with questions. Wilson-Barnett (1996) has argued that, for many, sex is 'a closed and private topic although it may be of vital importance to an individual's quality of life'. This lack of awareness among health workers is evident from the lack of available research into the role of sexual guidance and is an area that needs to be given attention.

At the beginning of this chapter, Jane expressed her satisfaction at working with this client group. Working with the elderly continues to be a popular area of health care and is likely to be a rapidly developing area for new research and interest as the number of elderly people increases.

# References

Age Concern (1992) *Comments on the Health of the Nation White Paper*. Age Concern, London.

Argyle, M., Martin, M. and Crossland, J. (1989) Happiness as a function of personality and social encounters. *Recent Advances in Social Psychology: An International Perspective*. Elsevier Science Publishers, London.

Bee, H. (1994) *Lifespan Development*. Harper Collins, New York.

Bleathman, C. and Morton, I. (1992) Validation therapy: extracts from 20 groups with dementia sufferers. *Journal of Advanced Nursing* 17, 658–66.

Busse, E.W. and Wang, H.S. (1971) The multiple factors contributing to dementia in old age. In *Normal Ageing 2* (E. Palmer, ed.). Duke University Press, Durham, North Carolina.

Department of Health (1992) *The Health of the Nation*. HMSO, London.

Eisdorfer, C. (1983) Conceptual models of ageing: the challenge of a new frontier. *American Psychologist* 38, 197–202.

Erikson, E. (1959) *Identity and the Life Cycle*. International Universities Press, New York.

Erikson, E.H., Erikson, J.M. and Kivnick, H.Q. (1986) *Vital Involvement in Old Age*. Norton, New York.

Feil, N. (1982) *Validation: The Feil Method*. Edward Feil Productions, Cleveland.

Goudie, F. and Stokes, G. (1989) Understanding confusion. *Nursing Times* **85**(39), 35–37.

Henwood, M. (1992) *Through a glass darkly: community care and elderly people*. King's Fund, London.

Kliegl, R., Smith, J. and Baltes, P.B. (1989) Testing the limits and the study of adult age differences in cognitive plasticity of a mnemonic skill. *Developmental Psychology* **25**, 247–56.

Laurer, J.C. and Laurer, R.H. (1985) Marriages made to last. *Psychology Today* **19**(6), 22–26.

McDermott, S. (1995) The health promotion needs of older people. *Professional Nurse* **10**(8), 530–33.

Neugarten, B.L. (1974) Age groups in American society and the rise of the young old. In *Political Consequences of Aging* (F.R. Eisele, ed.). American Academy of Political and Social Sciences, Philadelphia.

Neugarten, B.L. (1975) The future of the young old. *The Gerontologist* **15**, 4–9.

Olds, J. (1995) Strategies of care for patients with old age. *Professional Nurse* **10**(9), 585–87.

Sammartino, F.J. (1987) The effects of retirement on health. *Social Security Bulletin* **50**(2), 32–47.

Sternberg, R.J. (ed.) (1990) *Wisdom: Its Nature, Origins and Development*. Cambridge University Press, UK.

Raynor, E. (1986) *Human Development*. Routledge, UK.

Rikli, R. and Busch, S. (1986) Motor performance of women as a function of age and physical activity level. *Journal of Gerontology* **41**, 645–49.

Rimmer, L. (1982) *Reality Orientation: Principles and Practice*. Winslow Press, Bicester, UK.

Verhaeghen, P., Marcoen, A. and Goossens, L. (1992) Improving memory performance in the aged through mnemonic training: a meta-analytic study. *Psychology and Ageing* **7**, 242–51.

Willis, S.L., and Nesselroade, C.S. (1990) Long term effects of fluid ability training in old age. *Developmental Psychology* **26**, 905–10.

Wilson-Barnett, J. (1996) Commentary: facing up to taboo subjects: elder abuse and sexual counselling. *Nursing Times Research* **1**(6), 429.

# Further reading

Bond, J. and Coleman, P. (eds) (1990) *Aging in Society: An Introduction to Social Gerontology*. Sage Publications, London.

Issacs, R. and McMahon, C. (eds) (1996) *Care of the Older Person: A Handbook for Care Assistants*. Blackwell Science, Oxford.

# Chapter 7

# Approaches to the Care of the Adult with Mental Health Disorder

This chapter will explore how the three therapeutic approaches described in this book can assist health care workers to understand disordered behaviour and how to apply specific skills.

For most carers, their own apprehension about dealing with mental health disorder improves when relationships are formed with the patients, talking and 'getting to know them' as individuals, as was the case with Margot in the following account. 'Getting to know' someone takes time and energy. It often involves dismantling preconceived notions and perceptions about others and gradually allowing oneself to get closer to the other person. The context of the professional or therapeutic relationship means that clear boundaries dictate how close the relationship becomes. In the field of mental health work the relationship clearly becomes a very important one in terms of intimacy within the relationship. The relationship requires a level of genuineness in order for the therapeutic process involved in the closeness to benefit the patient. The 'intimate relationship' between health worker and patient is often cited by nurses in the mental health field as the main reason for working in this area (Moir and Abraham, 1996). In this context 'intimacy' is regarded as a relationship whereby the carer develops a close rapport with the patient and is concerned with getting to know how the person thinks and behaves and to offer close support.

*Margot – second-year student nurse*

'Like most of the students I was really worried about having to deal with mental illness. A colleague of mine had recently finished working in an orthopaedic care area where a patient became very depressed and ended up "hearing voices". I remembered her describing feeling "totally inept" and also embarrassed during the first few days. This is all I could think about whenever I had to care for anyone with a psychological problem. Despite these early misgivings, I did discover that this is a very important and rewarding area of care.

Thinking back, part of my anxiety was that I felt more "exposed" when caring for this group of patients – less able to use the barrier of my "role" to keep some space between us. I felt I had to rely more upon my relationship with the patient and be in closer proximity to the patient's personal life. This can be intimidating at first and much more intimate. I recall myself dreading that I would be asked questions that would show up my total lack of knowledge about their conditions. All the other permanent staff of the unit seemed much more relaxed and friendly but I did not want to appear totally incompetent to them.

It was therefore with some relief that I found myself starting to feel more relaxed after a few weeks. My fears started to diminish as I got to know the patients and staff better. I suppose there are a number of specific fears that most health professionals have initially about psychiatric conditions. In addition to the fears about not knowing "what to say to the patient" and feeling deskilled in the new situation, there is the fear of violence and of being involved in a threatening situation of some kind. In any clinical area there is a potential for verbal or physical aggression to be displayed and there is a fear of this being increased in psychiatric settings. The perceived fear of aggression therefore needs to be put into perspective. In psychiatric care areas this is handled and contained by the staff very quickly and proficiently. It is therefore possible to experience more incidents of psychiatric disorder, or of disordered behaviour, in many non-mental health areas, for example accident and emergency departments, intensive care areas.

My relationships with patients who suffered mental illness were more intense and I really appreciated the care with which I was treated by all of the mental health team. One difference for me was the regularity with which the "supervision" was arranged. This gave me the opportunity to discuss with my supervisor all aspects of care, including my fears and apprehension. Although a bit wary of disclosing anything personal at first, I soon realised that this was an expectation of all staff working in the unit, and when I observed even the senior staff discussing their own difficulties I was able to feel safe enough to join in. This form of clinical supervision had been very different from the usual "mentoring" experience I had encountered in previous placements.

Understanding and awareness of possible underlying explanations for the patient's behaviour helped me to feel more confident about how to approach each person and even at times gave me a better idea of what to say'.

Margot raises a number of serious concerns in the above account. Many students who work in mental health care settings fear physical violence and having to deal with hostility. Another common fear is concerned with aptitude and the ability to 'know what to say' to distressed patients, and being 'seen to be competent' by senior colleagues.

## Psychodynamic approaches

The most common feature in any psychiatric disorder is *anxiety*. An essential skill is therefore learning how to remain calm and instill calmness and confidence in the patient. This is not always easy to accomplish; however, there are a number of key elements which help to achieve this.

Anxiety consists of physiological and psychological components. There are clear biological elements to the experience of an anxious state; the American physiologist W.B. Cannon (1932) described the response as the *'fight or flight' mechanism*. This is where the 'autonomic' part of the nervous system prepares the body for immediate response in reaction to a perceived threat. The autonomic nervous system is concerned with stimulation of adrenaline which raises blood pressure and increases tension in the muscular system (Fig. 7.1). However, this discussion is primarily concerned with how anxiety affects the individual emotionally. The perception of an 'anxious state' has been described as a:

'continuum of emotional reactions to stress or fear which vary from abject terror to mild apprehension'.

(Rycroft, 1968)

Clearly one person's fear can be another's excitement, for instance the most frightening ride at the funfair is sought out by some and totally avoided by others. Thus the experience of anxiety is more than biological. Psychological concepts such as trust, safety, security and risk appraisal also play a significant role.

In the psychodynamic approach, behaviour is considered as being largely unconscious. The main focus of the carer's work, is to involve the patient in developing *insight*, that is, an understanding of the possible

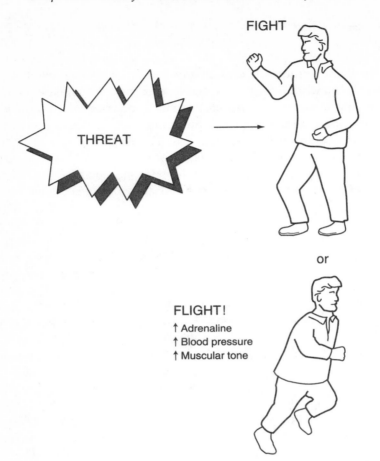

**Fig. 7.1**   The autonomic 'fight or flight' mechanism.

underlying causes of the behaviour. For example, a person who is very frightened may unconsciously repress his fears and deal with the fear by denial and projection on to others. This may manifest itself by the patient refusing to acknowledge his own condition and focusing on other people's disorders rather than consider the full weight of his own. This 'defence' can be helpful to the patient, allowing him time to come to terms with the situation. However, there will be a moment when the carer has to help the patient to come to terms with reality. In some mental health conditions there may be hidden 'benefits' in adopting the symptoms; however, the reader's attention is again drawn to the fact that this will be an unconscious process.

*Clinical example*

Mrs Doreen Dixon was referred to the psychiatric services by her doctor. For the past 3 years she had become increasingly dependent on her husband and children, more recently becoming totally housebound. This involved a fear of leaving the house, even to open the front door to anyone. For the past few weeks, Doreen has been living as a virtual self-imposed prisoner.

Her two children, both teenagers (aged 15 and 13 years), do the shopping for the family on the way home from school but have found their mother's behaviour to be more and more unpredictable. Recently Doreen has been phoning the school to ask for information, such as shopping lists, to be passed on to the children.

Doreen's husband, Bill, has been troubled by persistent phone calls from his wife and now refuses to discuss anything with her when she phones him at work. Usually the calls are to ask him what time he will be home from work and, although at first he tried to reassure his wife, this did not work, as she would phone him back again within 10 minutes. Bill confided a long-standing tension between them and that 'his wife has always lacked confidence in herself'.

Doreen is now unable to go anywhere and becomes panic-stricken at the thought of going to the shops or leaving the safety of her home.

The above situation reveals a classic description of the misery experienced by those suffering from *agoraphobia*. In this condition the patient becomes increasingly cut off from natural human interaction, as in Doreen's case, becoming totally dependent upon the family.

The psychodynamic approach begins by looking for 'clues' about what may be happening in the relationship. The aim is to understand the ways in which 'power' is maintained and managed within the family relationships. The possible advantages or *'secondary gain'* may give clues to what Doreen may gain by the symptoms and provide an overall understanding of what is actually going on in this family.

There are difficulties in the relationship between Bill and Doreen and they are no longer able to discuss their concerns with each other. In such situations there is often a real or imagined threat to the relationship which is being *denied* by either one, or both, in the relationship. Doreen feels anxiety at her perceived inability to alter her situation, which has become increasingly worse. Feeling unable to resolve this situation in any way, the anxiety becomes *repressed*, or 'pushed out of mind'. Through the process of *displacement* (see Chapter 2), Doreen attempts to reduce her level of anxiety by transferring or displacing her anxiety on to another situation. In this case she develops an incapacitating fear of leaving the house. The '*gain*' to be achieved through this mechanism is thus twofold. First, Doreen develops a 'condition' in which she is able to communicate her vulnerability. The family have to take care of her, do the shopping, show concern, and Doreen gets indirect attention. Second, she is able to communicate her vulnerability to Bill through the disorder. Such behaviour may also be an attempt to regain his care and attention and make it very difficult for him to leave her. The very nature of the agoraphobic symptoms means that Bill spends more time with her, as she is unable to be on her own for very long and cannot leave the house. It is important to reiterate that Doreen is not aware of using these mechanisms in any conscious way and the symptoms are real to her.

Freud argued the universal use of 'ego' or mental defence mechanisms to reduce anxiety, and that this is how the pressures of daily living are managed. Problems arise when, as in Doreen's case, the attempted solution is an unhealthy one and gradual incapacity develops. (The reader is reminded of a fuller account of psychodynamic defence mechanisms given in Chapter 2.)

Psychodynamic theorists, such as Freud and Erikson, have argued that everyone has to resolve critical events related to their physical, psychological, social and spiritual development, and that this occurs throughout life. The natural transitions required for growth from one stage of life to another, for example from adolescence to adulthood, trigger the crisis. Some cultures have very precise gateways between stages. Such 'rites of passage' allow each stage of life to be entered with clearly delineated rules. However, in western societies, transition between the stages of life may be more confused. Freud focused on childhood up to adolescence, and did not discuss development beyond this stage. Jung (1968) focused more on the 'second half' of the human life-span, particularly on old age, which will be considered in the next chapter.

Erikson (1950) proposed three stages during adulthood:

- young adulthood
- middle age
- old age.

Within each period of time, the individual has to deal with change. Dealing with the crisis created by the changes requires the use of mental defence mechanisms to defend against the stress and struggle of development. At these change periods an increase in anxiety will occur if other events coincide, such as employment, unemployment, marriage, divorce. All are more likely to occur more frequently in the adult phase of life. How a person reacts to each of these events will vary. As described earlier, some people thrive on stressful situations, while others become quite unwell. If stress continues, it can cause psychological disorders, which bring the sufferer into contact with the health services. Doreen was clearly having to deal with two children who were now into their adolescence, with all the changes to their re-accommodation of her role towards them. Clearly she was having difficulty within her own relationship with them and with her husband, which the symptoms helped her to avoid facing. The reader may note that the term 'illness' is being deliberately avoided in this context, as many of the psychiatric conditions that require therapy do not fit the usual definition of illness, which normally implies an underlying abnormal pathology.

## Intimacy versus isolation

In adult life, Erikson (1950) suggests a transition from adolescence to young adulthood in the stage described as *intimacy versus isolation*. This stage is characterised by a gradual move towards mature commitment to others. In a relationship this may mean sacrificing one's own needs and the development of intimacy. Intimacy here means the capacity towards understanding one's own needs, personality changes and the achievement of reasonable self-confidence. This is essential before the individual can really be committed intimately to a relationship with another person.

Conflicting feelings often exist towards the demands of an intimate relationship with another person. This stage is a time of experimentation during which an intense desire to be independent and to act as a mature adult gradually develops. Competing with the desire to be independent are feelings of wanting to be loved and cared for. The young adult may deal with this by withdrawing from what he perceives as feeling too 'exposed'. Early adolescence is usually a time of profound embarrassment and in extreme moments social contact is difficult to deal with (see Chapter 4).

In clinical depression an underlying mechanism is *introjection*. In an extreme case the individual internalises all that he perceives wrong with himself and the world, in a negative way. The process of 'introjecting' is a natural developmental phase and is often manifested by periods of morose indifference to others and self-absorption. Unhealthy self-absorption due to this mechanism can occur in some patients in response to severe stress. An example of this occurs where the patient has an unhealthy belief in his own self-importance, not in any boastful or obvious way, but at a more profound unconscious level. The individual may feel that he is the only person who can solve or resolve others' problems, and believes himself as the 'centre' of events, unhealthily omniscient.

According to Freud, this mechanism is present in every person; however, as the 'ego' develops and the individual matures, he begins to gradually accommodate a more balanced perspective, based upon reality, rather than an idealised *ego-orientated* view of the world. It is the mechanism which many health workers can identify with, as they come into careers with a better ability than most to communicate and be special for someone else. Many carers, for example, put their own needs last. Such characteristics are very noble until they become exaggerated and under stress can become unhealthy.

### 'Narcissistic' behaviour

In some instances the behaviour can become very unhealthy, and such individuals demonstrate *narcissistic* behaviour. This feature of personality behaviour was first described by Freud who used the Greek myth of Narcissus as an analogy to explain such self-orientated behaviour. Narcissus fell in love with his own reflection. The individual who invests greatly in an image of 'self' as being singularly important in the lives of others may be commendable, but this can also have a very damaging effect when it becomes all-pervasive – particularly so when there has been some history of childhood trauma, when narcissistic feelings are essentially about gaining transitional security.

Narcissistic actions often arise from a damaging past history, such as childhood abuse. In such situations a fundamental anger exists which has been unconsciously internalised, denied, and only leaks out during times of extreme stress. It is often characterised by apparently self-destructive behaviour, such as abuse of alcohol or other substances.

Destructive angry behaviour may also be directed towards an intimate partner and may include cheating or dishonesty, which may appear out of character. Such behaviour can be understood in terms of a barrier being created by the individual, due to the damaged past. This blocks or splits off the person's healthy development. The individual is in a state of crisis, not able to commit himself to a relationship and not easily able to find a solution.

The role of the carer is to build a relationship where the patient can be challenged and confronted with the internal anger. The therapeutic skills require gentle confrontation of the 'split-off' behaviour. The aim is to enable, at first, awareness, and then understanding of the detrimental effects, both to self and others. Behaviour based upon narcissistic anger can occur at any time in adult life but may be particularly triggered at the time of divorce, or around mid-life, particularly for men. There are often tragic histories of failed or part-failed relationships with intimate partners, which often motivate the person to seek help. The skills involved in caring for such self-destructive behaviour are the ability to set very firm limits, in terms of what behaviour has to change; careful exploration of the underlying anger that is the real cause of the narcissistic behaviour; helping the patient to fully acknowledge the extent of his behaviour and the damage it continues to cause him and others.

Recovery is often very dependent upon the individual being able to trust the carer enough to explore very painful internal feelings and memories, and thus often requires a consistent, lengthy time period. When the patient is motivated to change, it is possible for positive change to occur.

## *Dealing with transference reactions*

As in all approaches, the skill of 'active listening' is a factor in the development of trust. This is the precursor to being an effective helper. The therapeutic skills are built upon this foundation and rely upon the ability to understand the *transference* reactions that are likely to occur, and deal with them in a direct way. Transference, as noted earlier (see Chapter 5), is a 'key' psychodynamic concept, consisting of a tendency to 'transfer' feelings, either positive or negative, to the other person in the relationship. It offers an explanation for how it is possible, on first meeting another individual, to experience either warmth or unaccountable dislike. Such feelings may not be due to anything the person has said or done during the brief encounter.

In the same way that certain smells or music can be very evocative, so transference phenomenon can be equally powerful in creating feelings that affect the relationship. A common process would be for the client to transfer feelings of 'authority' to the helper, effectively treating her as a parental figure. If this is allowed to develop, the patient may become increasingly dependent, effectively *regressing* and in extreme circumstances, becoming totally dependent on others and acting in very 'childlike' ways towards staff.

Patients can very easily become 'dependent' upon the caring staff, particularly with all their attendant anxiety due to concerns about their illness, being away from loved ones and being in a strange environment. Awareness of the transference reactions is thus an important part of the therapeutic alliance between helper and patient – remaining alert to anger, tension, or exaggerated affection, which may all indicate trans-ference reactions.

## Guilt, rituals and obsessions

Regression, as the previous account has described, is where the indivi-dual exhibits behaviour from an earlier stage of development, for example behaving in childlike ways. It is commonly due to increased stress and anxiety and acts like an unconscious 'safety valve', letting off steam. Many adult disorders, such as *obsessive–compulsive* disorder, have their origins in the magical quality of childhood thinking, where in order to exert some 'control' on the world and reduce anxiety, rituals are performed. Such simple activities like stepping over the cracks in the pavement, or throwing 'salt over the left shoulder', 'touching wood' to avoid disaster, are all examples.

Children often show mild compulsive or ritualistic behaviours as a means of gaining security. For instance, the small child may insist on parents checking under the bed and in the wardrobe, to check for 'monsters', before settling down to sleep. Such activity usually increases when the child is anxious. In adulthood, obsessive personality characteristics can develop into maladaptive behaviour when the stress is perceived to be overpowering for the individual. 'Compulsion' refers to the need to perform an action repeatedly. This is illustrated in the clinical examples which follow.

### Clinical example (a)

Ms Ashman had been admitted to an acute medical area following a referral from her GP. A single woman of 30 years living alone, she had been experiencing night sweats during the past few weeks, had lost weight and was found to have generalised swelling of lymph nodes. An intelligent woman, she feared that she had cancer. Ms Ashman descri-bed herself as a very 'organised' person who 'could not stand anything out of place in her house'.

Shortly after admission she became very concerned about personal hygiene and staff noted that she would spend at least an hour washing in the morning, midday and evening. While this did not in itself present any abnormal pathology, staff became concerned that the obsessive nature of the activity was very much connected with her anxiety. One of the staff was able to talk about her fears with her in a more direct way. After a few days the rituals began to reduce in frequency.

### Clinical example (b)

Mrs Gordan had been admitted to the mental health unit following a domiciliary visit by the local mental health team. Her general practitioner had treated Mrs Gordan for obsessive–compulsive condition for the past 2 years with varying degrees of success; however, the current exacerbation was creating intense problems for both Mrs Gordan and her family and they agreed to a visit from the team and to her subsequent admission.

Mrs Gordan's behaviour consisted of ritualistic and repetitive handwashing: in fact, so repetitive that her hands were raw and sore from repeated rubbing. Her family reported that she was now unable to leave the bathroom, feeing compelled to wash her hands all day. They reported that on 4 days in a row they had left the house in the morning and returned from work or school in the evening to find her very distressed and still at the sink.

Mrs Gordan was aware that her behaviour was obsessive and disordered but felt unable to stop the behaviour. The washing served to reduce her anxiety and if she did not give in to the intense compulsion to wash her hands she felt 'panic-stricken, dirty, and guilty'. In order to feel 'clean' Mrs Gordan washed her hands in a specific order, starting with each fingernail, finger, palm and back of the hand, finishing with a final wash of the whole hand. If the sequence was broken, she felt compelled to start again. Soon the washing with soap did not seem enough and she used new 'scrubbing brushes', and the bristles made her hands red raw. She now surpassed the rigour of a surgeon before an operation in her need to get clean, but her actions were insufficient to her and became a form of self-inflicted punishment.

The conditions which have just been described are often associated with feelings of *'guilt'* and may be interpreted as an attempt at absolution – the washing away of guilty feelings, perhaps for some past indiscretion. Other 'ego defence mechanisms' feature in the psychopathology of such disorders and include *displacement*, the transferring of an anxious internal state of mind on to a more outward object – in the previous examples, on to excessive washing in an attempt to reduce the intensity of feelings. Unfortunately, this does not happen and the individual may become increasingly distressed and the behaviour becomes disruptive to everyday living.

The skills needed to assist in such conditions require an understanding of the possible underlying pathology. The patient requires constant reassurance and encouragement, the aim being to assist the patient to 'let go' of the intense fear associated with not performing the rituals. Even though the patient understands the futility of his actions, they serve to reduce the anxiety. Temporary relief occurs as a result of performing the actions, never satisfying the need for long, hence the repetition. The carer's task is to break the patient from the obsessive action. Essentially her role is to act as a 'nurturing parent', using the 'transference reactions' that are created in the relationship. The aim is to create a 'safe' and 'containing presence', for example a person who can be trusted, who understands the misery of the patient's position and who offers care.

The next stage is to explore the underlying anxiety in more detail. There is likely to be much resistance to the unfolding of these feelings, which have been repressed and locked away from conscious appraisal for a long time. Again the critical skill is for the helper to maintain a consistently safe environment and to be consistent in her reassurance and presence. It would be non-therapeutic to begin such work knowing that in 3 weeks' time she will be away on leave.

### Denial, projection and paranoid states

In an attempt to deal with anxiety that is perceived as overwhelming, the individual may use the mechanisms of *'denial'*. This is frequently manifested in the patient who 'refuses' to acknowledge the reality of a situation, for instance, in a serious illness.

A *psychosis* refers to a state of mind where the individual represses events that are occurring in everyday life, and loses contact with reality. A main feature of such conditions is the presence of *delusional ideas*. These are fixed false beliefs that are impervious to any attempt of reasoned argument by others. A person with delusional ideas 'believes' in their internal view, no matter how irrational it seems to outsiders. Denial is a feature in the development of the delusional system.

In many clinical settings the carer may see patients with *paranoid beliefs* that others are against them or trying to harm them. This form of behaviour utilises the mechanism *'projection'* as the underlying dynamic. Projection is the process of attributing unacceptable parts of the self, which are 'denied', and perhaps disliked, on to others. Feelings such as suspicion are personal characteristics or personality traits. Suspiciousness is often the basis of jealousy. Accusations about fidelity in a relationship may come from the individual's own internal aware- ness of his potential to be 'unfaithful' – a lack of trust in himself, resulting in feeling unable to trust others. Such individuals are constantly jealous of their partners.

In more serious cases this becomes the basis of paranoid delusional states, where the individual may fear he is being poisoned or under threat. Caring for individuals in this condition requires a whole team approach. Assessment of the possible danger that the patient may pose to others is important. Hostility is a main feature of paranoid states, as the patient attempts to defend against their perceived danger. The role of the team is to present a consistent view of reality, to reassure, taking care to understand that for the patient the fear is real, without colluding with the delusional ideas.

## Affective states

Denial forms the first attempts, by the individual under stress, to deal with perceived pressure. The more unhealthy mechanisms form part of the unconscious attempt to live with the stress. In Chapter 2 the mechanism known as *'reaction formation'* was discussed. This is where the individual expresses behaviour which is the opposite of their internal feeling. This mechanism forms the basis of the 'manic- depressive' or affective disorder, where the main characteristics are extremes of mood swing from elation to profound depression. This condition is also referred to as 'bi-polar disorder', which is a reference to the swing from two poles of mood (see Fig. 7.2). A mild analogy of this process is how many people react when their mood is low, by attempting to 'jolly' themselves out of that frame of mind.

*Hypomania* is a more extreme reaction, where there is no conscious effort to 'pull oneself' out of a bad mood. The mechanism is a totally unconscious attempt by the mind to 'deny' the psychic pain. Patients with fully established hypomanic states demonstrate restless activity and may be a threat to themselves because of this. It is often possible to uncover deep sadness and depressed thinking – the 'tear of the clown' appearing on a falsely smiling face. According to the psychodynamic

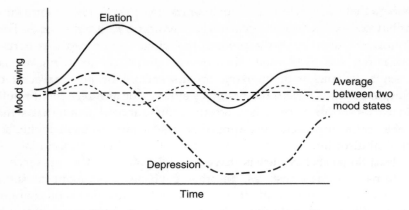

**Fig. 7.2**   The graph demonstrates how, for most people, there is some swing either side of the average between the two extremes (. . . .). However, some individuals swing more erratically, and may require treatment for depression (— · —) or, in some cases, abnormal elation (—).

approach, such behaviour may be seen as an attempt by the mind to deny the pain.

The skills required to care for such a disorder consist firstly of very close observation in the acute stages, to ensure the client does not become a danger to himself or others. There is a high risk of suicidal attempts, particularly as the patient begins to recover, when there is sufficient awareness within the person of their condition, often associated with sadness and shame. Care consists of support during the manic phase and, as the client calms down, the ability to help reduce the anxieties through patient education. In many clinical settings patients may become unnaturally cheerful, or giggly, the so-called 'manic-defence' against their fears.

A different perspective will now be discussed, by reviewing behavioural approaches to care.

## Behavioural approaches

Although the behavioural approach has been largely replaced by more recent developments in the therapeutic arena, such as cognitive behaviour therapy (Barker, 1990, p. 44), the principles of the behavioural approach remain the same for the basis of understanding clinical applications. This approach accounts for all behaviour as a result of learning and therefore abnormal or undesired behaviour can be treated using relearning techniques. Such an approach can only be applied to individuals who have the potential for learning new behaviours. Thus children are usually very adept at responding. The longer the pattern of behaviour has been established, the longer it normally requires to change. Patients with memory impairment are usually excluded on clinical grounds because retention of events, and the necessity to build upon recall of success, are essential for success. Other than this, behavioural approaches are applied across a wide spectrum of ages and clinical disorder.

Traditional behaviourists have no tolerance of the presence of 'internal mechanisms' as in the psychodynamic approach. In behaviourism, the therapeutic process is only concerned with changing observable behaviour. For example, Skinner (1979) has argued that 'the inside of an organism' is irrelevant as it cannot be studied 'scientifically'. Skinner, was one of the most ardent behaviourists and argued that an individual's behaviour was totally influenced by the environment.

In an earlier clinical case example, Mrs Doreen Dixon's disorder was explored. The following discussion will apply a strictly behavioural therapeutic approach, and thus enable the reader to make a comparison between the two ways of 'approaching' the main features of the condition.

The aim of the treatment is to change undesirable behaviour so that Doreen becomes free of the constraining effects of her behaviour. A thorough assessment would be made by the 'therapist' who is a health worker, trained in behavioural therapy techniques (Marks, 1985). Starting from a relationship of trust and confidence, the carer will seek consensual agreement on a detailed plan for recovery. This would form the basis of a 'contract' between the patient and the helper. This is usually a 'hierarchy' of tasks which gradually approximate the desired behaviour. For example, in Doreen's case the plan would be as follows.

- Walk to the front door and open it.
- Next stage – walk out of the door and then back in.
- Progress to the front gate of the house and back inside.
- Next stage – to the street and then to the end of the road.

Each stage would increase when the preceding task had been success-fully accomplished. The agreed objective may be to get to the shops and actually buy some items, say a grocery trip. At each stage the helper is supportive, gives verbal encouragement and non-verbal support through touch, holding of hands, arms or whatever gives the patient added confidence. The patient must be able to trust the helper, who does not do anything other than what is written and agreed in the 'contract', in other words no sudden or unexpected demands or requests. During the planning of the treatment, Doreen would have been taught relaxation exercises, which consist of deep breathing, how to relax shoulder and neck muscles, and how to prevent *hypocapnia*, using a paper bag. (Hypocapnia, in this context, occurs when the client is very anxious and over-breathes very rapidly. The effect of this hyperventilation creates feelings of faintness which obviously increase the panic. The patient is usually very frightened, pulse rate is rapid and over-breathing will lead to collapse due to imbalance of oxygen and carbon dioxide levels. Breathing into a paper bag assists in recovery through re-inhalation of the expired air, which is higher in carbon dioxide content. This helps to restore the imbalance more rapidly.)

Doreen would have been taught how to record her anxiety levels by indicating on a scale of 1–10. When the ability to utilise the relaxation techniques has been practised with some proficiency, and the helper feels that sufficient rapport has been established with Doreen, the process begins. On each successful completion of a set task, for instance getting to the front gate and back with reasonable control of the anxiety level, Doreen is *rewarded*. This is usually profuse praise and encouragement, but may also be rewards that have been negotiated beforehand and which are meaningful. This may be anything from chocolates to a bunch of flowers from the family. The family members are usually involved in the treatment, so that they are party to the process and can share in the development of a comprehensive treatment plan.

A successful outcome is measured by Doreen reaching the agreed treatment goal, and treatment will continue until this objective has been reached. In Doreen's case it means being able to visit the local shops on her own. This outcome usually brings some increase in self-confidence and raises self-esteem. It does not, however, investigate the reasons for the condition developing in the first place, or the possible tension or dynamics involved within the family. Behavioural approaches are only concerned with the objective measurement and evaluation of what can be observed and quantified.

This example describes just one behavioural method. However the principles involved in this method have common denominators. For health professionals, the relationship and development of trust must be present before any hope of recovery is possible. Reward for appropriate behaviour is fundamental. Where undesirable behaviour occurs, this is ignored. The objective is to attempt to 'extinguish' the pathological and encourage healthier behaviour through giving more attention to what is required. The principle involved in this process is the technique of *operant conditioning*, outlined by Skinner (1953; see Chapter 2). Skinner proposed the method called *successive approximation* or '*shaping*'. This technique is the underlying behavioural explanation for the method used to treat Doreen's condition. It is the process of giving immediate rewards to behaviours that get closer and closer to the desired objective.

At times it may be necessary to implement *negative reinforcement* as a means of encouraging the desired behaviour. This does not mean, as the name suggests, a painful or punishing technique. Negative reinforcement is the removal of a 'non-rewarding' situation or stimulus. It is often used in child and adolescent areas to reduce antisocial or aggressive behaviour in disturbed children. The 'time-out' technique is an example of this method. In this situation, when the child misbehaves he is removed to his room and is not allowed to play with the other children. When he behaves, he is told that he can return. Thus the removal of the 'time-out', that is, time away from play with others, is the negative reinforcer, which hopefully will change the behaviour.

Behaviour therapy is often used to treat phobic conditions such as Doreen's agoraphobia and other anxiety-related conditions. However, it has also been used with disturbed and institutionalised patients. In the latter instance, 'token economy' methods have been implemented, where the 'rewards' are the actual payment of tokens which can be later exchanged for goods or privileges. Additionally, behavioural approaches have been applied to the treatment of anxiety states in children and adults, personality disorders and severe psychotic conditions.

Behavioural methods have, as outlined at the beginning, been subject to considerable criticism for imposing a rigid deterministic regime on to human behaviour (Schultz and Schultz, 1994). Critics argue that individual actions cannot always be controlled by reinforcement, although pivotal concepts of learning, reward and reinforcement remain valid as components of the therapeutic method still used in many settings.

## Person-centred approaches

The person-centred approach is more concerned with how the environment affects the individual – factors affecting the perception of self-worth and self-esteem. Both self-worth and self-esteem are implicated in maladaptive methods of coping. Rogers' (1951) early work focused on early family development, particularly family environment and social interactions occurring between family members and the effects of the family culture upon the individual. He attempted to observe and study how the child made sense of these influences and made sense of the world. He explored concepts such as 'self-understanding' and self-awareness and found that it was the latter state of 'self-insight' which was to become a more powerful predictor of later behaviour.

Rogers later founded the 'client-centred' approach, based upon the view that all individuals in the progress of growth and development are motivated towards a need to enhance self-potential. However, this tendency may become *negatively affected* in early childhood, when self-regard and self-confidence become blocked. For example, if a mother is able to demonstrate total and 'unconditional' love for the child (what Rogers describes as *'unconditional positive regard'*, see Chapter 2), the child will grow in a positive way and develop an inner sense of *positive self-regard*.

In Doreen's condition (see clinical example), the ability to view herself and the world positively becomes a source of increasing anxiety. Doreen may have always held a low regard for herself in the past and tended to narrow experiences in her life that could have helped her to grow emotionally. For example, meeting other people, or taking risks socially, would have been avoided because of her poor view of herself. The fear of meeting others often stems from feeling that others will not want to know them, or that they will have 'nothing to say'. This results in a general opting-out of social engagements, constantly narrowing the social field. Avoidance works as a temporary strategy, until extra stress creates self-doubt and problems begin to develop. In Doreen's case it may have been a fear that she was no longer loved or needed by her family.

Rogers has developed the concept of *incongruence*. This is a discrepancy between a person's *self-concept*, or how they perceive themselves, and the actual reality of their situation. Doreen's situation may be viewed as a worsening of her negative self-concept: 'My family does not need me, then other people will not love or like me, because I am a worthless person and I am fearful of going out and meeting other people . . .'. A person's ability for healthy adaptation is dependent upon the ability to perceive situations objectively and to view alternative ways of coping with personal stressors. Believing in one's ability to see the world as it really is rather than as it may at times feel, which is often very different. According to Rogers, people are *freely open* to all experiences when they possess a healthy self-concept, or where the person is able to take 'knocks' because they possess a sense of 'balance and self-esteem' to get over a personal trauma (Rogers, 1983).

Ill health and hospitalisation obviously have an effect upon a person's view of self. Clearly there will be differences depending upon the severity of the condition; however, any illness that causes even temporary incapacity, alters self-concept for a while. For the carer, the interpersonal skills involved are constructed around the three central pillars of this approach: the ability to show warmth, positive uncondi- tional regard, and to be genuine. The aim is to achieve positive change, which means the encouragement of 'growth and development' away from the disordered behaviour patterns (Bertin, 1990). Trust has to be built so that the patient feels confidence in the carer's ability to help the development of self-regard. This means that at times the patient's self- belief will need to be challenged, by working through the origins of negative beliefs.

French (1994) suggests that loss of confidence is the most frequent accompaniment of the anxious state, and describes the skill of reassuring the patient as a 'purposeful attempt' to restore confidence. The skills of reassuring consist of a number of sub-skills. These include:

- offering explanation and education (Wilson-Barnett, 1979)
- use of touch and physical contact (French, 1994)
- helping clients to verbalise fears and encourage catharsis (Wilson-Barnett and Carrigy, 1978)
- challenging or gentle confrontation, and offering support (Heron, 1990).

## *Patient education*

Giving information to patients about their health is a potentially powerful way of giving reassurance; however, the carer must be aware that giving too much information may have the opposite effect and raise anxiety levels. Therefore it is important to be vigilant and certainly explain everything that is happening, but check the patient's responses for signs of agitation.

Generally, education and explanation are essential to allow the individual involvement in their care and allow decisions to be made. The critical skill is to ensure that encouraging involvement is performed when the patient is able to do so. Patient education includes teaching techniques to reduce anxiety, such as deep breathing and relaxation exercises. Awareness of prescribed medication and the likely side-effects of these substances is also fundamentally important.

## Touch and physical contact

Human contact is a very potent reducer of anxiety, especially during times of stress and worry. However, many health professionals are fearful of close contact with patients (MacLeod-Clark, 1981). Clear boundaries and definitions of how physical contact can used therapeutically is required by the health worker in order to clarify the use of techniques such as massage. There is now considerable research to substantiate what is already intuitively known by mothers, that contact is vital for normal healthy development (Harlow and Harlow, 1962; French, 1994). Touch is effective in providing comfort (Stevens, 1975) and has a calming effect. Bennett and Braun (1986) warn that as it is such a 'potent' therapeutic tool, it must be treated with respect. Not all patients will find being touched reassuring, some clients perhaps perceiving the movement as provocative or threatening (Jacobs, 1988).

However, for most people, techniques such as gentle massage, holding the worried patient's hand, a steadying hand on a person's arm or shoulder, are all effective ways of reassuring a tense and anxious person. Increasingly, health care workers are becoming trained in the use of 'essential oils' and aromatherapy techniques as alternatives to, or used in conjunction with, prescribed analgesic chemotherapy. Such methods, when used appropriately, have very powerful effects and are being increasingly requested by patients. Very distressed and anxious clients are particularly helped and such remedies can produce sedation without the usual harmful side-effects of conventional treatments. The author can recall working with a charge nurse in an acute psychiatric unit, who always advocated supervised baths for tense patients. A very warm bath sprinkled with oils and bath salts nearly always worked well, relaxing tension and helping patients to sleep, while also aiding the reduction of prescribed medication.

## Encouraging 'catharsis'

Catharsis refers to the release of tension and emotions. Helping patients to express their worries and concerns is an important element of reassurance (Heron, 1990; French, 1994). Techniques include encouraging the patient to verbalise concerns and giving permission for the person to cry. A typical situation is where the patient is obviously working hard to suppress tears. The carer can collude with this suppression, motivated by an attempt to avoid embarrassment. Alternatively, the carer can stay with the patient in their distress, encouraging the release of feelings. The carer needs to take the risk of saying 'It's alright to cry' or give permission for the patient to release upset and tears, supporting him by remaining present.

### Confrontation

According to Heron (1990) this skill is the most inappropriately applied by the majority of health professionals. Confronting, in this context, does not mean aggressive challenging. Rather, it is the skill of gently giving feedback, in a direct way so as to challenge the beliefs, or behaviour. The relationship between carer and patient has to be well-established, with sufficient rapport, before such interventions can have any therapeutic effects. Care is very necessary when dealing with suspicious personalities or patients with paranoid delusions.

Patients in intensive care areas may become confused and disorientated due to a number of factors which become exacerbated by the surrounding environment. Where such confusion leads to delusional thinking, the carer can attempt to deal with the situation by empathising with the way the patient feels, acknowledging the anxiety and fear generated by the delusional idea, *while not colluding with* the delusional content.

The person-centred approach can be summarised as an attempt to allow the individual to develop self-confidence and self-esteem. This is carried out by utilising the therapeutic relationship between the patient and carer and adopting an open, accepting and non-threatening approach. Where behaviour requires to be challenged or confronted, the approach continues to value and accept the *person* while rejecting the behaviour. Change is facilitated through being supportive and 'present' for the patient. This helps to reduce anxiety and allows the patient's own coping mechanisms to be explored, challenging unhealthy views of the self.

## Conclusion

The health professional working with a patient's mental health disorder, uses her relationship as the main therapeutic tool. This chapter has attempted to explore the three approaches, applying them to common situations. In so doing it has sought to contrast the differences in approach offered by each method. In practice, parts of each approach are used when working with patients, as indicated earlier in this book. Each approach does, however, have its own unique elements and these have been highlighted in this chapter.

Research evidence now being collected on the effectiveness of therapeutic approaches indicates the need for carers to be critically aware of the differences between each approach, and to develop more research into which method to adopt in specific disorders; for example, when to use a more directive, behavioural approach and when to allow the patient to be more active in their own care. This is to be preferred to applying them in a haphazard way.

# References

Barker, P. (1990) Cognitive therapy model: principles and general applications. In *Psychiatric and Mental Health Nursing: Theory and Practice*, Chapter 3 (W. Reynolds and D. Cormack, eds). Chapman and Hall, London.

Bennett, G. and Braun, M.D. (1986) *Treatment of Multiple Personality Disorder*. American Psychiatric Press, California.

Bertin, D.A. (1990) The Rogerian client-centred model: clinical applications. In *Psychiatric and Mental Health Nursing: Theory and Practice*, Chapter 15 (W. Reynolds and D. Cormack, eds).

Cannon, W.B. (1932) *The Wisdom of the Body*. Norton, New York.

Erikson, E.H. (1950) *Childhood and Society*. Norton, New York.

French, P. (1994) *Social Skills for Nursing Practice*, 2nd edn. Chapman and Hall, London.

Harlow, H.F. and Harlow, M.K. (1962) The effects of rearing conditions on behaviour. *Bulletin of Menniger Clinic* **26**, 213–24.

Heron, J. (1990) *Helping the Client*. Sage Publications, London.

Jacobs, M. (1988) *Psychodynamic Counselling in Action*. Sage Publications, London.

Jung, C.G. (1968) The archetypes and the collective unconscious. *Bollingen Series*, Vol. 20, 2nd edn. Princetown University Press, Princetown, USA.

MacLeod-Clark, J. (1981) Nurse–patient communication: an analysis of conversations from surgical wards. In *Nursing Research: Ten Case Studies in Patient Care* (J. Wilson-Barnett, ed.). John Wiley, Chichester.

Marks, I.M. (1985) Psychiatric nurse therapists in primary care. Research report, Royal College of Nursing, London.

Moir, J. and Abraham, C. (1996) Why I want to be a psychiatric nurse: constructing an indentity through contrasts with general nursing. *Journal of Advanced Nursing* **23**, 295–98.

Rogers, C.R. (1951) *Client-centred Therapy*. Houghton Mifflin, Boston.

Rogers, C.R. (1983) *Freedom to Learn in the Eighties*. Merrill, Columbus, Ohio.

Rycroft, C. (1968) *Anxiety and Neurosis*. Penguin, Harmondsworth.

Schultz, D. and Schultz, S.E. (1944) *Theories of Personality*. Brookes–Cole Publishing Company, California.

Skinner, B.F. (1953) *Science and Human Behaviour*. Free Press, New York.
Skinner, B.F. (1979) *The Shaping of a Behaviourist*. Knopf, New York.
Stevens, R. (1975) Interpersonal communications. In *Social Skills for Nursing Practice*, 2nd edn (P. French, ed.). Chapman and Hall, London.
Wilson-Barnett, J. (1979) *Stress in Hospital*. Churchill Livingstone, Edinburgh.
Wilson-Barnett, J. and Carrigy, A. (1978) Factors affecting patients' responses to hospitalisation. *Journal of Advanced Nursing* **3**, 221–28.

# Further reading

Freud, S. (1901) The psychopathology of everyday life. In *The Standard Edition of the Complete Psychological Works of Sigmund Freud*, Vol. 6, (ed. J. Strachey). Hogarth Press, London.
Freud, S. (1940) An outline of psychoanalysis. In *The Standard Edition of the Complete Psychological Works of Sigmund Freud*, Vol. 20, Hogarth Press, London.
Jacobs, M. (1986) *The Presenting Past*. Open University Press, Oxford.

# Chapter 8
# Approaches to Cultural and Spiritual Care

This chapter will deal with two areas of care that have become increasingly important elements of holistic patient care. The world has seen a recent need to come together in the expression of deeply felt emotion. The death of Diana, Princess of Wales moved individuals from a variety of cultural and spiritual ideologies all around the world, with a fundamental need to share their grief. The intensity of this need has surprised many commentators, however it clearly reveals deeper internal needs within all of us. Within health care, concerns about human spirituality and awareness of cultural difference, have been given insufficient attention (Dobson, 1991; Stoter, 1995).

Thus these two areas have been chosen for discussion in this final chapter as they present continuing challenges to health care staff and occur frequently enough in everyday practice to warrant discussion of more effective therapeutic management.

## Transcultural care

Jet travel now allows the experience and ease of travel to a significantly larger group of people and the world is a smaller place than it once seemed. This means that there is much more exposure to other cultures and customs and, for health workers means that they will increasingly meet patients from cultures other than their own. There is a saying that travel either 'broadens the mind or increases the prejudice'. For some health workers there is little understanding of the needs of people from other countries. Assumptions are therefore made in often complete ignorance of other cultures and practices, which leads to stereotyping behavioural traits of others who are different.

Margaret, a second-year student nurse, recalls working with a patient from Greece. She was on holiday in this country and was admitted as an emergency to the medical care area during Margaret's placement there.

'I was aware of how frightened the woman was at the time of her admission. She had been admitted for investigation of suspected "diverticulitis" (inflammation of a blind sac or pouch which buds out from the wall of the large bowel). This lady was on holiday visiting her son in the UK and had never been out of Greece before. She spoke very little English and it was very difficult to explain to her what was happening at first. Her daughter-in-law, who is English, came in with her as the patient's son was at work and attempts were made to contact him. Her daughter-in-law spoke a little Greek. However it was very hard for her to translate the explanations given by the doctor. It was unclear whether the attempts to explain were making things worse, as the daughter-in-law, also looking anxious, struggled to find the correct translation.

I can remember this lady was very constipated and the medical staff wanted her to have an enema. It was decided to wait for the son to arrive so that he could give a better explanation to his mother. He arrived 3 hours later, having travelled directly on hearing the news. On his way he had obviously collected other members of the family and about 15 people suddenly surrounded the patient's bed, all talking in excited mixes of English and Greek. They wanted to know what was happening, all at the same time, and I found it difficult to calm them.

They were clearly anxious, but realised that they were beginning to get in the way of our attempts to care for the patient and they left the son to explain to his mother what was happening.

The lady stayed in the ward for several days as there was a fear that she may have developed localised ulceration as a complication. She was treated with antibiotics and pain relief. We discovered that many members of her family had travelled with her from Greece and that this was her first time out of her country. She was a deeply religious person of Greek Orthodox religion and the family arranged for a priest to come in to give her communion. Again we tried to accommodate the family and the patient with as much privacy as possible, which was not easy in the traditional setting of the medical hospital ward. We managed to move her bed into a corner of a bay where there was an empty bed alongside. This enabled the family to join in the service and we were able to pull the curtains around the two bed cubicles to offer some seclusion.

A different set of cultural traditions was operating in relation to this woman's care. I had never been to Greece, however was now experiencing the extended family in action, as large groups of people, all related in some way to the patient, would visit and sit around her. They would all bring their food and on one occasion all sat eating their lunch. This was in stark contrast to the other patients on the ward. It was a very pleasing experience for me to see how caring and supportive a large family could be. This lady received many visitors and I thought how much this raised her morale'.

Transcultural care is an attempt to address the reality that society is becoming more and more multicultural due to increased travel and mobility, and that the health worker needs to be aware of transcultural issues in their practice. This does not mean developing an 'encyclopaedic knowledge' of the world's cultures (Dobson, 1991), but rather to be aware of key principles of working within a multicultural context. Culture in this section refers to the socially inherited beliefs and understandings that are carried by a society. *Culture* can be defined as the 'way of life' of an entire society. This includes code of manners, dress, language, rituals and systems of belief (Jarry and Jarry, 1991). Culture is often used to refer to ethnic groups. An *ethnic group* is a group of people sharing the same distinct origins and therefore the same culture.

Another term used in this context is *race* which refers to the biological origin of the person. It usually refers to differences such as skin colour and bone structure and includes cultural differences. Dobson (1991) argues that while the 'scientific validity' of the term 'race' is of some questionable value, it is a powerful 'social labelling device'. Dobson highlights the conclusions of the Black Report (DHSS, 1980, p. 17) which exposes race as being an important 'dimension of the inequality in contemporary Britain'.

Transcultural care refers to the ability to offer skilled and culturally aware health care. Where the carer and patient come from the same cultural group, the care is provided on an *intracultural* basis. Where the carer and patient are from different cultures, then it becomes *intercultural*. *Transcultural* care is therefore the ability to work interculturally (Dobson, 1991).

One of the pioneers of transcultural care is Madeleine Leininger (1988). Leininger worked as a psychiatric clinical nurse specialist in the 1950s, with disturbed children. At that time the psychodynamic approach was the predominant approach to the care of the child and was used to plan most nursing interventions. She observed that patients in her care came from a wide variety of cultural backgrounds, which affected all of their everyday activities. The psychodynamic explanations were insufficient to explain the diversity of behaviours and she

turned her attentions to *anthropology* for a better under
Anthropology is the study of human societies, focusing on cust
approach has been particularly influential in the development ~~or North~~
American nursing, which has led to a growing awareness of the cultural
dimension in nursing and to a growing literature on this subject.

At the heart of such an approach is the need to be aware of barriers
either emanating from the carer herself, or from the restraints of the
'external' situation. Providing comfort, empathy, nurture and 'succour'
remain at the centre as key constructs of care.

The basic interpersonal skills begin with very careful listening and
attention to non-verbal behaviour. Even when the language is not
understood, there are universal signals and communications such as
laughter, sorrow, or pain, which can be very obvious. Empathy is the
ability to understand what the patient may be experiencing (discussed in
Chapter 5). In the previous account, Margaret could fully appreciate the
anxiety the patient was feeling and the probable frustration. Most of us
have been on holiday in a foreign country and can recall the embarrassment and effort required simply to ask for everyday items. In this
instance, she was able to easily imagine how the patient must be feeling,
what being in hospital, in a strange country must feel like for her.
Building empathetic skills are clearly going to help in any interaction;
where there are differences in cultures, it encourages a sharing of
intercultural disparities. This begins with an active attempt to build
understanding.

This understanding has been described as *'transcultural reciprocity'*
(Dobson, 1989, 1991). The development of interpersonal skills begins
with assessment. The carer begins to work with the family and relatives
of the patient, putting together a composite understanding of the
cultural differences, beliefs and background events that may contribute
to the patient's health. If the patient cannot speak English, a translator
can be called in. This may be a relative of the patient; however, most
health teams have a list of individuals and the languages they speak,
who can be quickly called in to assist communication. Additionally text
'translators' are available, either electronic dictionaries or printed
directories of common languages and terms.

Collecting this information together has to take place as quickly as
possible and therefore direct questioning of relatives for culturally
relevant information is necessary. Brownlee (1978) has argued that
collecting this information is vital to transcultural care; for example,
knowing about fasting and prayer which, if ignored, can cause increased
and unnecessary anxiety.

Dobson (1991) suggests three 'pivotal' concepts involved in inter-cultural situations:

- caring
- collaboration
- creativity.

## Caring

Culturally relevant care means including an awareness of the patient as a 'cultural being', respecting the values and traditions of the patient. In an attempt to communicate clearly, the carer may employ psychodynamic ideas, such as how mental defence mechanisms and anxiety are 'managed' by the patient. Care has to be taken that such interpretations are legitimate. This means being able to check them with the patient and this requires the clear use and understanding of language. Thus there is a real criticism that psychodynamic understanding can only be really helpful when there is a thorough knowledge of the patient's culture.

Behavioural techniques such as observation and participation, or a focus on behaviour, may seem more 'objective'. However, it has also been pointed out that behaviour is very related to settings and cultural influences. Peacock (1986) has argued that although health workers may be keen observers, 'patterns of behaviour' are of more value than individual snapshots, or isolated responses by a person which may mean very little unless an understanding of the context in which the behaviour has occurred is known and understood by the observer. The crucial factor is for the carer to resist making instant judgements even though this may be very difficult, as most appraisals about others tend to be unconscious. However, an attempt can be made to understand the patient's background and customs, before making interpretations about behaviour.

## Collaboration

Thus the next concept, that of collaborating, can be aimed for. This effectively means attempting to work together with the patient, being open and clarifying the cultural background, making an attempt to overcome barriers and obstacles to care.

## Creativity

The final concept of multicultural care is to integrate the patient's cultural traditions into the planning and delivery of care. Margaret described in her account how difficult it was to accommodate the needs of her patient within the limitations of a medical care area, which was not designed to give appropriate multicultural care. However, with thought and ingenuity, compromises can be negotiated.

It is possible to use a *cultural assessment guide* as a check-list. One example is Brownlee's *Cross-cultural guide for health workers* (1978). Although now 20 years old, it still provides a very helpful guide, covering communication, language, religion, the family, and health beliefs and practices. Another guide which can assist care workers is Leininger's (1988) *sunrise* model, so described because what are considered cultural issues are set out in the shape of a semi-circle in the diagram (see Fig. 8.1). This model provides a useful framework to address key interpersonal areas of care because they are seen as 'influencing care patterns through language and environment' (Dobson, 1991). In assessing an individual's cultural needs, attention is given to concepts such as 'technology, religion and philosophical factors, kinship

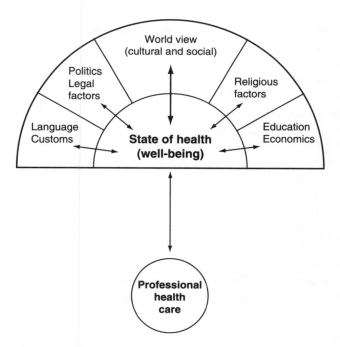

**Fig. 8.1** Adaptation of Leininger's 'sunrise model' (1988). An arch is depicted which represents cultural dimensions. The factors, such as politics, religion and education, which are within the semicircle, will all influence health care.

and social factors, values, education, politics, and economic factors'. Interpersonal communication is based upon an awareness of the need for three actions from the care giver:

1. cultural care preservation
2. cultural care accommodation
3. cultural care repatterning.

*Cultural care preservation* is the attempt by the carer to assist and facilitate the patient of a particular culture to maintain or preserve the beliefs and systems of his culture in order to recover from illness.

*Cultural care accommodation* is where the carer can assist the patient to adapt or change part of their belief in order to achieve a satisfactory health status. This may have only limited potential in some instances, and is likely to be more successful when explored with the patient's family or significant contacts.

*Cultural care repatterning* involves assisting patients to actually do more than adapt, and to change their cultural beliefs and consequent lifestyle, through education. These changes, however, must be culturally meaningful to the patient and support healthy life styles.

The person-centred approach to health care may be a more appropriate method of providing transcultural care. The approach is based upon assessment of day-to-day need and attempts to understand the changing health needs as they emerge. As stated in several parts of this book, the important aspect is to use the most appropriate and informed way of understanding and responding to the patient. This may mean a combination of all three approaches.

Many racial and cultural minority groups experience powerlessness when faced with health care services where most organisations are 'unicultural' in nature (Dobson, 1991). Often only tacit acknowledgement of the need for informed multicultural practice is in evidence. However, the realities of being increasingly in contact with other cultural traditions means that health care workers are themselves seeking to deliver culturally sensitive interpersonally skilled care. This section can only raise very brief awareness of some ways of enabling this to occur. The reader is asked to consider their own level of awareness and practice, and seek to improve care in this area.

## Spiritual care

Health care workers are often unsure about including considerations of 'spiritual care' in their practice with patients. Until recently the domain of spiritual care was considered to be the main province of the hospital chaplain. Part of this is due to the ambiguity and confusion that has existed about what spiritual care really means. It is often assumed that it is the same as religious care (Stoter, 1995). More correctly, spiritual care refers to the search for meaning in life, a unifying force that integrates the physical, emotional and social dimensions of a person's sense of self (Socken and Carson, 1987). Spirituality is not necessarily concerned with religious beliefs or rituals. It is therefore just as appropriate a concern for the agnostic or atheist.

Johnson (1997) considers that spiritual distress is accompanied by a number of concerns. These include:

- feelings of guilt
- feeling a lack of purpose or meaning in life
- alienation from others or from God or other higher powers
- conflict between religious or spiritual beliefs and the prescribed health care plan
- lack of forgiveness of self or significant others.

Spiritual crisis is accompanied by a complex array of feelings which often include despair, a sense of emptiness, anger, discouragement, resentment, ambivalence and a fear about life's meaning. Such feelings are often present when a person suffers from a chronic or terminal illness. Frequently a patient will express a tremendous burst of anger and sadness, racked with a mixture of these feelings, and asks why 'this has to happen to me'. A range of defence mechanisms are then introduced by the individual to deal with the enormity of the situation.

Frequently the carer's role becomes confused at this stage. Many consider it more appropriate to leave the patient, to allow space for contemplation, a hope perhaps that relatives will be able to help 'pick up the pieces' in a more effective way. However, to the contrary, the carer's role is to remain and make a more informed assessment about whether this is the case. Remaining present and giving support and reassurance, the carer is required to stay with the patient. This may allow the patient to cry, to release pent-up emotion, or provide the opportunity of talking more openly about fears. Carers often attempt to stop the crying by giving insincere or unrealistic reassurance. It is very tempting to want to do this, to relieve the pain. However, this often leaves the patient feeling isolated by their condition, or just increases the fear and loneliness which is often experienced by patients. The security for the patient is often simply having someone near and to feel less alone.

Establishing clear eye contact is important. Many individuals unwittingly avoid any prolonged eye contact when they feel embarrassed or when having to deal with taboo issues such as the fear of dying. Non-verbal communication, particularly facial expression and eye contact, is important in this context and carers need to become more aware of how they communicate during such encounters and attempt to focus on attempting to be more relaxed and 'engage' with the patient in a more confident way. Even if the carer is new and does not feel very confident, maintaining good eye contact and observing the patient's responses is a way of improving interpersonal skills.

Person-centred approaches focus on the importance of assessing human need. Maslow's hierarchy of human needs (Maslow, 1970), for example, explores the need for the individual to work towards 'self-actualisation', a need for achievement of self-potential and spiritual fulfilment. Self-actualisation represents a person's ultimate pursuit of self-fulfilment and peace of mind. This is fundamentally important and achieved through striving to interact in the world in a meaningful way. One of the reasons that unemployment has had such a tragic effect on the human spirit has been the sense of hopelessness it has created in a society that still values work as a means of providing a sense of identity. For instance, people still ask you 'what you do' at social events as a means of communicating and getting to know you. Presumably this is still much easier than asking 'who you are!'.

It may not be obvious to a patient who is suffering and in distress to be fully aware of what their spiritual needs may be. The language used in the intervention has therefore got to be straightforward. The skill is to appraise the importance of any consideration associated with spirituality, which helps to give comfort and security. The role of health worker is to instil hope and attend to needs that are not always expressed. A patient and his family may have never really contemplated this need, until stricken with illness or grief.

Spiritual care is an area where there are very few straightforward answers to the questions (Stoter, 1995). Sometimes it may be appropriate to ask the patient (or a relative) about their beliefs. Occasionally it helps to make the issue explicit – simply asking a direct question about whether a person has a belief in God or in some higher being and showing a willingness to open up this area for discussion. This may be helpful for the patient who may have been troubled by such thoughts, but unsure how to raise them. Interventions need to be appropriate for the patient's understanding. The carer can therefore be alert to the patient's ability to understand what is being discussed, that is, make judgements about the person's ability to think abstractly and under-stand deeper meanings (Peterson and Nelson, 1987).

Health carers have to deal with the basic and fundamental aspects of life and death. Many situations bring the need for spiritual support into sharp focus. Working with the dying patient and the relatives, the mentally ill, dealing with patients who are attempting to cope with actual or potentially disfiguring surgery, patients recovering in the coronary care or intensive care unit – all have to deal with the physical and psychological shock of their condition, and undergo a traumatic re-evaluation of their life. It is mostly the case that all patients who emerge from some life-threatening or severe illness, often do so with a changed perspective on life. Learning how to help in this re-evaluation is part of the total process of caring and yet it is, sadly, neglected by health care staff.

Working with patients from different cultures also presents challenges for the health worker. The importance of spiritual beliefs and customs varies considerably. For example, a patient, Mr B, believed that he had an 'evil spirit' within him and this was the cause of a severe infection of an abdominal wound. In this instance Mr B also had considerable guilt about a past affair and had not been able to forgive himself. He believed that the infection was a 'punishment' for his act. Staff were able to explain the reasons for the infection and that such occurrences unfortunately occur to people. This was reinforced by the whole team.

His wife had died in a car crash several years ago and he ruminated on his indiscretion without really feeling able to talk openly to anyone about it. He related this story to a 'key' nurse who was caring for him during his admission. She had established a relationship with him and the story tumbled out one day, when he became tearful after the nurse had changed a messy abdominal dressing. The nurse later established that he was a Christian, who felt very ambivalent towards 'God' since his wife had died. The nurse suggested to him that he might find it helpful to talk to the hospital chaplain. This offer was turned down by him at first; however, he later asked to see him. He was able to tell the chaplain how he felt and confide in him about his past indiscretion, which seemed to provide considerable comfort and relief to him.

Caring for the spiritual needs of the patient helps significantly in the patient's peace of mind and in their recovery from ill health. While this awareness has been raised in this section as a 'separate' part of the overall care, it is of course an integral element of the full and total care of a person. Therefore carers are required to include this consideration as an essential part of the skilled interpersonal care.

### Consideration of the carer's own spiritual needs

It is very difficult for any health professional to be effective without being aware of their own interpersonal and spiritual beliefs. To be able to understand a patient's spiritual needs, the carer has to assess her own needs (Johnson, 1997, p. 165).

One study of nurses' ability to provide spiritual care, found that it was either very superficial, with a narrow range of skills, or was delivered at a deeper personal level. The main difference between the superficial and deeper abilities was the nurses' own awareness of personal spiritual beliefs and values. Often these had developed as a natural consequence of life experiences, having grown through a crisis in their own lives (Ross, 1994).

To summarise, health carers have to clarify their own attitude and position towards spiritual elements of life. Within society, the pluralistic confusion concerning differences between religion and spiritual issues 'muddies the water'. This often leads to feelings of inadequacy and lack of confidence about providing this care. The concerns are related to not knowing how to deal with patients' needs at this level. Perhaps a fear of raising the subject leads to an avoidance of spiritual questions in the assessment of a patient's total needs. The carer may feel that it is a 'private concern' (Granstrom, 1985). If a patient senses this, he also may avoid increasing the carer's apprehension and a collusion of silence develops, creating a spiritual 'black hole' – a vacuum, which assumes the patient is only concerned with their physical or psychological health care.

Attention to the patient's spiritual needs is part of the 'holistic' approach to health care (Fig. 8.2), involving consideration of the physical, psychological, social and *spiritual* needs of the patient.

## Conclusion

Spiritual and cultural care are two interlinked and often neglected areas of interpersonal care. Stoter (1995) argues that a relationship between the carer and patient that is based upon 'equality, mutual commitment ... and good communication' is likely to be personally rewarding for the carer as well as the patient.

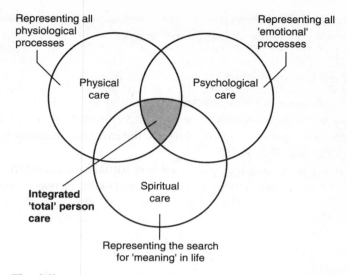

**Fig. 8.2**   The different aspects of care that are integrated to provide holistic, 'total person' care.

This requires the development of a partnership based on trust. For those with a particular faith, the health worker is required to be open to the significance and importance of this belief in the delivery of care. Thus spiritual and cultural should be assessed and integrated within the care plan in an appropriate way.

# References

Brownlee, A.T. (1978) *Community, Culture, and Care: A Cross-cultural Guide for Health Workers*. Mosby, St Louis, Missouri.

DHSS (Department of Health and Social Security) (1980) *Inequality in health*. Report of a research working group, chaired by Sir Douglas Black. DHSS, London.

Dobson, S.M. (1989) Conceptualizing for transcultural health visiting: the concept of transcultural reciprocity. *Journal of Advanced Nursing* **14**, 97–102.

Dobson, S.M. (1991) *Transcultural Nursing*. Scutari Press, Royal College of Nursing, London.

Granstrom S.L. (1985) Spiritual nursing care for oncology patients. *Topics in Clinical Nursing Care* **5**, April, 39–45.

Jarry, D. and Jarry, J. (1991) *Collins Dictionary of Sociology*. Harper Collins, London.

Johnson, B.S. (1997) *Psychiatric Mental Health Nursing: Adaptation and Growth*, 4th edn. Lippincott, Philadelphia.

Leininger, M.M. (1988) Leininger's theory of nursing: cultural care diversity and universality. *Nursing Science Quarterly* **1**(4), 152–60.

Maslow, A.H. (1970) *Motivation and Personality*. Harper & Row, New York.

Peacock, J.L. (1986) *The Anthropological Lens: Harsh Light, Soft Focus*. Cambridge University Press, Cambridge.

Peterson, E.A. and Nelson K. (1987) How to meet your client's spiritual needs. *Journal of Psychosocial Nursing* **25**, May, 34–39.

Ross, L.A. (1994) Spiritual aspects of nursing. *Journal of Advanced Nursing* **19**, 439–47.

Socken, K.L. and Carson, V.J. (1987) Responding to spiritual needs of the chronically ill. *Nursing Clinics of North America* **22**(3), 603–11.

Stoter, D.J. (1995) *Spiritual Aspects of Health Care*. Mosby, London.

# Chapter 9
# Conclusions: An Eclectic Approach

We all live and work in a world surrounded by objects of all shapes and sizes, and yet are fascinated by other people. Witness the behaviour of others (including ourselves) in airport departure lounges and in train stations and it becomes clear that we all like to observe the activity of other people, no matter how hard we try to remain unnoticed by those we are observing.

This book builds upon this natural curiosity and applies it to the context of the caring professional, focusing on three main approaches to understanding human behaviour: the psychodynamic, behavioural and person-centred approaches. Each theoretical approach has been described and explored within the context of developmental stages of the life-span. Additionally, because other important areas of concern for practitioners transcend the human life-span as discrete sequences in life, cultural, spiritual and mental health issues have been discussed in separate chapters.

Each chapter has opened with a narrative from a different health carer, such as a nurse, occupational therapist or medical student. The predominant experience described has been from the nursing profession which reflect the writer's own background; however, the theoretical ideas and their application have been explored because they are common to *all* who work in the caring service. Increasingly, exploring the care of patients from a multi-professional perspective is being recognised as a priority in planning health care (Barr, 1996). Practitioners are already aware of the importance of working more collaboratively in understanding the unique skills that different professional groups have to offer in consideration of the patient's total care. The attempt in this book to use examples of narratives from the carers who do work together to achieve this aim, is a further attempt to develop such links. However, in a book of this size it is not possible to include all carers who contribute.

The three theoretical approaches chosen have been an implicit component of much of the teaching of interpersonal skills in health care practice during the past decade. The practitioner who understands which theory or collection of ideas underlies her interpersonal awareness, is likely to be more clinically effective (Dryden, 1984). Chapter 2 presented the three approaches which were then explored in ways in which the practitioner may be able to apply the ideas in her everyday practice. Common experiences have been chosen as they present a possible way of interpreting the theory in practice.

In everyday practice the carer is, of course, likely to apply the best of whatever approach fits the situation. Each approach is an attempt to understand the human condition and develop interpersonal skills that are effective in improving communication between the carer and the patient. The skilled carer is one who is aware of the approach they use in their own practice. The skilful practitioner uses an underlying knowledge of theory in order to inform her practice. To the casual observer this appears effortless. Rather like the experienced car driver being unconsciously aware of how they use the pedals, they will apply what is the most likely to benefit the patient. However, on reflection, skilled practice can be analysed and critically appraised according to an underlying method. Critical appraisal means being able to reflect on what was actually happening, what theoretical approaches were being used and how to evaluate the outcome. It is only possible to assess this with a knowledge of what the theories represent and the differences between them. This book provides the carer with frameworks for critical examination.

Each of the approaches described has developed and evolved over a period of almost 150 years and continue to be refined and reworked as new knowledge adds to the debate. Each approach will have its own advocates and critics and this has been discussed in various parts of the book. Similarly, the 'life-span' approach to human development has its own detractors, a point made at the beginning. The most obvious criticism of the life-span approach is that it artificially compartmentalises human growth and development into stages that only exist as 'averages' of human performance. Such critics would prefer to see human life as a more dynamic flow of activity which cannot be pinned down easily to chronological periods.

While all of the above arguments have validity, the purpose of this book is to explore common situations with which health carers can readily identify. An *eclectic* approach takes the 'best' from each of the approaches and applies it to the clinical situation. No single approach is likely to be able to explain the full range of human behaviour and each has advantages and disadvantages as an interpersonal technique. Dryden (1984) refers to 'hat-rack' eclecticism when the practitioner tries various methods in a haphazard way. There is evidence that being more aware of technique is of benefit to the patient when applied within psychological counselling (Dryden, 1984).

It is hoped that readers will be able to develop critical awareness of each approach, and appraise it within the context of their own practice. Further, that this will enable the carer to develop interpersonal skills which are not haphazardly applied, but well understood in terms of their theoretical and practical value. This will allow the carer to work eclectically in an informed and critical way.

Being interested in the behaviour of other people and wishing to work to help them achieve a state of well-being involves three important prerequisites: to listen in an active way, to be aware of relevant theoretical ideas which improve interpersonal skills, and to be able to apply these in a sensitive way. Hopefully, readers will find the ideas expressed in this book helpful in being able to achieve this.

# References

Barr, H. (1996) Ends and means in interprofessional education: towards a typology. *Education for Health* **9**(3), 341–52.

Dryden, W. (1984) *Handbook of Individual Therapy in Britain Today*. Harper & Row, London.

# Index

active listening, 85
active parenting in childhood, 45
adolescence
   in childhood, 46
   and health, 63
   suicide, 64
   sub-culture, 64
affective states, 137
ageing, effects on society, 107
aggression, 73
agoraphobia, 129
ambivalent feelings, 6
anal stage of development, 38
anger, 34, 74
anorexia, 37, 64, 69
anthropology, 151
anxiety, 6, 13, 92, 127–30
anxiety, symptoms of, 14
assertiveness, 5, 95–9
attachment theory, 42–7
authoritarian personality traits, 18
autonomic nervous system, 127
autonomy, 41
avoidance, in children, 46

barriers to communication, 7
behavioural approach
   assessment, 73, 98
   theory, 20–24
   in childhood, 53
   in adolescence, 70
   in adults, 95–9
   in the elderly, 113–15
bereavement, 110
Black Report, 150
blaming, as a defensive response, 94
biological changes in adolescence, 63
bi-polar disorder, 137
bonding, 42, 43
Bowlby, J., 42
bulimia, 69

catharsis, 16, 144

childhood, 32–58
children's fears in hospital, 34
child death, 55–7
classical conditioning, 1, 22
cognitive behaviour therapy, 138
collaboration, in intercultural care, 152
communication
   definition, 4
   in children, 35
   types, 94–6
compromise, as an interpersonal skill,
   98
compulsive behaviour, 134
conditioned reflex, 21, 22
confidence, lack of, 5
confrontation skills, 77, 145
conversion, 68
counter-transference, 88
crisis periods in development, 40–42
crying in childhood, 35, 36
cultural assessment, 153
culture, 64, 148–51

defence mechanisms, 15–20
defensive behaviour, 39, 94, 95
delusions, 136
dependency, fear of, 118
denial, 19, 45, 129, 136
depression, 119, 137
de-skilled, 3
disowning, as a defence against
   anxiety, 19
displacement, 18, 19, 68, 111, 129
dreams, 11
dying
   child, 32, 55–7
   adult, 121–2

eating disorders, 37, 68
eclectic approaches, 30, 162
ego, 12, 13
ego-orientated, 132
ego defence mechanisms, 15–20

emotional 'holding', 54
emotional security, 122
empathy, 29, 78
Electra complex, 39
ethnic group, 150

facial expressions in the child, 35
family centred care, 45–7
fight/flight mechanism, 127
forgetfulness, 15, 16
free choice (in philosophy), 10
Freud, S., 9, 10, 16, 20, 25
    criticism of, 40
Freudian slips, 12
'fruit machine', as example of operant
        conditioning, 24
frustration-aggression hypothesis, 73

genuineness, 29, 79
gerontology, 107
ground rules in health care settings, 6,
        54
guilt, 5, 134–6, 155

haphazard approaches, 9, 163
headache as symptom of anxiety, 14
health
    culture, 6
    in adolescence, 63
    in adulthood, 87
    in older people, 108, 112
    language, 6
    promotion in older age, 112
helplessness, 118
'here and now' theorists, 25
hierarchy of needs, 27, 28, 48, 118
holistic care, 1, 158–9
homeostatic mechanisms, 13
hope, instilling in patients, 93
hostility, 73, 90
humanism, 25, 28
hypomania, 137

id, 12
idealisation, 65
identification, 39, 78
identity, 66
illness, patient's experiences off,
        101–3, 118
imprinting, 42
information giving, 48
insight, 127
integrated care, 159

interpersonal skills
    definitions, 1, 4
    with patients and colleagues, 4
insomnia, 14
intimacy, 87, 131
introjection, 131

Jung, C., 20, 112
jealousy, 137

lack of confidence, 5
learnt behaviour, 20
limit-setting, 53, 70
listening, 7
loneliness, 155
loss, 14, 110

Maslow, A., 25, 118
massage, 93
masterbation, 65
maternal deprivation, 44
mechanistic view of behaviour, 10
mentor, 2, 3, 6
menstruation, 65
mood swings in adolescence, 62–6
mother–child bonding, 44
mourning, 110

narcissism, 132
negative reinforcement, 141
negotiation, 98
neo-natal intensive care, effects of, 36

obsessive behaviour, 39
obsessive-compulsive disorder, 134
observation, 119
Oedipus complex, 39
operant conditioning, 22
oral stage of development, 37

paranoid beliefs, 136
patient education, 143
Pavlov, I., 21
person centred approaches
    theory, 24–30
    in childhood, 47–53
    in adolescence, 78–81
    in adulthood, 99–103
    in the older person, 115–22
    specific person-centred skills, 28–30
phallic stage of development, 39
phobic reactions, 19
physiological needs, 28

placating, 94
plasticity, in human development, 114
play, 51–3
pleasure principle, 12
positive regard, 79
prejudice, 148
projection, 111, 137
psychoanalysis, 10
psychodynamic
   theory, 9–20
   in childhood, 47–53
   in adolescence, 66
   in the adult, 87–95
   in the older person, 109
psychosexual stages, 36
puberty, 65

questioning, 38

race, 150
relaxation skills, 93
rationalism, 10
rationalisation, 15
reaction formation, 17
reality orientation, 114–16
reassurance, 47, 93
regression, 18, 92, 133
reinforcement/reward, 23, 53, 72, 98
reminiscence therapy, 109
report/hand-over, 2
repression, 16, 68, 91, 129
resolution therapy, 116
restlessness, 14
rituals/ritualistic behaviour, 134

safety needs, 28, 48, 96
secondary gain, 19, 129
search for meaning, 155
self
   actualisation, 25–28, 115
   awareness, 67, 97
   concept, 25, 100–103, 142
   confidence, 5
   disclosure, 75
   esteem, 14, 18, 50, 115

identity, 14
separation, effects of in children, 45
sexual abuse, 40
sexual relationships in old age, 123
sexuality, development of, 39, 65
shaping, 141
silence, 5
Skinner, B.F., 22, 141
sleep disturbance, 119
social labelling, 150
social rules in health care settings, 6
splitting, 6, 17
spiritual beliefs, 157
spiritual care, 154
spiritual needs, 158
stimulus-response, 21
stress management, 93
sublimation, 16
suicide, 64, 87
suicide risk, 69, 119
superego, 12
suppression, 15
suspiciousness, 137

task assignment (as part of care
      planning), 6
technology, effects of, 36
total person care, 159
touch, 43, 143–4
transcultural care, 148
transcultural reciprocity, 151
transference, 88–92, 103, 112, 133
transitional stage, in adolescence, 63
trust, 29, 40, 137

uncertainty, 100
unconditional positive regard, 26, 142
uniforms, 7, 18

validation therapy, 114
verbal anger, (dealing with), 74–8

warmth, 29

yearning, in loss, 56